P9-BIM-571

ADRENALINE
DOMINANCE

A REVOLUTIONARY APPROACH TO WELLNESS

MICHAEL E. PLATT, M.D.

CLANCY LANE PUBLISHING
california

Clancy Lane Publishing
40493 Desert Creek Lane
Rancho Mirage, California, 92270

Glycemic index reproduced with the permission of Al Sears, M.D., from his website: www.alsearsmd.com.

Edited by Carolyn Bond, Editorial Arts
Designed by Jessica Stevens, www.design-savvy.com
Production: Chris Molé Design

Publisher's Cataloging-in-Publication Data
Platt, Michael E.
    Adrenaline dominance : a revolutionary approach to
    wellness / Michael E. Platt, M.D.
        pages cm
        ISBN 978-0-9776683-1-1
    1. Adrenaline--Health aspects--Popular works.
    2. Health--Popular works. 3. Hormone therapy--Popular works.
    I. Title.
    QP572.A27P53 2014   612.4'5
    QBI14-600094

Manufactured in the United States of America

10 9 8 7 6 5 4 3 2

NOTE TO THE READER

This book contains my own views and approaches to various medical conditions in men, women, and children. It is based on years of clinical observation and patient feedback, and is tempered by intuition and logic.

This book is not a substitute for any treatment prescribed by your physician. Any recommendations made in this book should be discussed with your physician, who can order any necessary laboratory evaluations and follow your progress, making adjustments in your treatment as required.

This book is not intended to be a medical textbook. The information contained within is to help you make informed decisions about your health. Hopefully it may provide you with enough information to guide you to wellness with the aid of your physician.

– Michael E. Platt, M.D.

I dedicate this book to my wife, Victoria,
who has never doubted me,
especially during those times
when I doubted myself.

*The doctor of the future will give no medicine
but will interest his patients in the care of the human frame,
in diet, and in the cause and prevention of disease.*

– Thomas A. Edison

CONTENTS

INTRODUCTION

This book introduces a revolutionary approach to treating many illnesses traditionally considered incurable simply by addressing their underlying cause. I have used this approach to help patients get well for two decades. However, this was not always the case. As is true for the majority of doctors, most of what I learned during my medical training was based on research provided by drug companies. By the time I finished my residency in internal medicine, I was convinced that no matter what the problem, a drug was needed to treat it. All this changed when I discovered the world of bio-identical hormones.

Bio-identical hormones have a molecular structure identical to those of the hormones the human body produces. Manufactured by drug companies such as Pfizer and Upjohn, with implicit FDA approval, they are then formulated by compounding pharmacies into creams, pills, troches, or suppositories. Since they are natural, they cannot be patented, which is why we don't see drug companies enthusiastically endorsing them.

Because hormones control every system of the body, they significantly affect how the body functions. Hormones out of balance can be responsible for many illnesses. Utilizing bio-identical hormones as a form of treatment thus offers an effective alternative approach to wellness. This is not "alternative medicine." It is traditional medicine using bio-identical hormones that have been in existence for over 70 years.

Over time, as I helped patients get better using this approach, I came to recognize certain similar symptoms as associated with a variety of disorders. These symptoms were all related to the excess of one particular hormone, namely, adrenaline—which led to my recognition of a condition I call "adrenaline dominance." At the same time, I discovered that bio-identical progesterone offers a natural, healthy, and effective way to help reduce excess adrenaline and also to help block its effects. By addressing the cause (i.e., high levels of adrenaline), rather than the symptoms, many conditions can often be eliminated, along with the medications used to treat them. Getting hormones into balance, changing the way people eat, and utilizing certain supplements can accomplish this.

The purpose of this book is twofold. First, I want to let patients who are struggling with health issues that never seem to improve know there is a different, healthier approach to getting them well. Second, I want to share what I have learned with other healthcare practitioners who are looking for a more effective way to treat patients and thereby possibly change, one by one, how individual physicians practice medicine. Hopefully, this book can restore the original goals many of us physicians had when we entered medical school, which were to help sick people get well and to help well people stay well. Hopefully, it will also reinstall the faith in medicine that patients used to have when doctors were highly respected.

Today, both physicians and patients have lost faith in the U.S. healthcare system, which has become a national disgrace. Even though the United States spends more money per capita on health care than any other developed country, we still have the highest incidence of diabetes, obesity, heart attacks, cancer, and infant mortality among all industrialized nations. The U.S. medical system is a multi-trillion-dollar-a-year industry thriving mostly on illness, not wellness. Drug companies benefit, as do hospitals and the providers of medical equipment. All the ancillary businesses involved with medical care provide millions of jobs and are the source of billions of dollars in tax revenues to state and federal governments from the sale of medical supplies. Is there any wonder that the incentive to change this system is in short supply? Not well publicized is the fact that health care is the number one budgetary item in most states. We can add to that the cost of Medicare, which is becoming an insurmountable financial burden for the federal government.

Drug companies greatly influence how physicians practice. Research conducted by these companies provides the basis for much of what is taught in medical schools, and many doctors are not comfortable making medical choices unless a drug company gives them direction. A simple example is the fact that many doctors never recommend supplemental CoQ10 when their patients are taking statin drugs because drug companies do not recommend it, perhaps to avoid liability issues. However, statin drugs prevent the production of CoQ10, which is essential for the function of muscles, including the muscles of the heart. With little or no CoQ10 in the body, muscle pain and even sudden death can occur.

Primary care physicians have traditionally formed the backbone of the medical field. Yet a recent poll of primary care providers indicated that, given the chance to do it again, 80 percent of them would not choose to go to medical school. Every year fewer medical students elect to go into primary care. The reasons are multiple: the long hours, the heavy patient load, and dissatisfaction with reimbursement of primary care compared to other specialties. At the time of this writing, implementation of the Affordable Care Act is unlikely to improve these figures.

Another factor contributing to the decline of primary care medicine may be the absence of the right tools to get patients truly well. If primary care practitioners were actually able to eliminate their patients' problems, they would receive plenty of positive reinforcement from a multitude of grateful patients. Instead, they are taught to prescribe drugs to lower blood pressure, drugs to lower blood sugar, antidepressants, sleeping pills, pain medications, plus others. As you will see in this book, excess adrenaline can be a significant factor in many of the problems for which drugs are prescribed. In fact, antibiotics are the only drugs that actually cure anything—all other drugs simply help patients to cope with their ailments.

This book calls into question many time-honored approaches to medicine. It proposes an approach that looks at causes rather than symptoms. It suggests that many conditions regarded as incurable can be eliminated without the use of medications, which often can be toxic. And it recommends bio-identical hormones and diet, rather than drugs, as treatment.

That said, this is not an anti-drug-company book. In fact, it is not anti anything. It is only promoting a different approach to practicing medicine that stands to provide greater satisfaction to both patient and doctor. Doctors who are comfortable relying primarily on guidance from drug companies must accept the fact that their patients will rarely, if ever, get cured. On the other hand, one of the rewards of the approach this book offers is the frequency with which patients will say, "Doc, in my entire life I've never felt so good."

Many of the ideas put forth here are likely to evoke resistance because they have not been subjected to the double-blind studies that have become the standard of present-day medical research. While double-blind studies can be great research tools, they are not perfect. It is widely recognized that their results can be skewed by the expectations of the researchers or to meet the needs of the funding drug company.

The ideas in this book are derived from a combination of observation-based and evidenced-based medicine. This is how most advances in medicine have been achieved throughout medical history: through observation followed by evidence to support that observation. Alexander Fleming's initial discovery of penicillin, for example, was purely observational. It took years before research revealed how and why penicillin works. Getting patients well should be the bottom line, whether or not there are journal articles to support the protocol. Progress in medicine has probably been delayed 50 years because "experts" have denigrated observation-based medicine to the category of anecdotal, that is, having no credibility.

The book begins with an explanation of adrenaline dominance, a discussion of the role and function of adrenaline in the body, and an overview of the basics of treating adrenaline dominance. The chapters that follow cover—with a nod to the title of Clint Eastwood's movie—the "good," the "bad," and the "ugly" effects of hyperadrenalism. I consider ADHD the "good" aspect of excess adrenaline, since it is associated with high intelligence, creativity, and success. Many famous and high-achieving people have ADHD. The "bad" forms of excess adrenaline include medical conditions that are more or less manageable. In the "ugly" category I have put conditions that significantly impact quality of life. These divisions are not meant to suggest that excess adrenaline is all good, all bad, or all ugly. Rather, a person with excess adrenaline will often have symptoms and conditions that fall into more than one of these categories. By lowering excess adrenaline a person can experience primarily the "good" aspect of adrenaline, that is, heightened intelligence and energy.

There is an extensive chapter discussing the specifics of treatment, including the use and dosing of progesterone, a diet for managing adrenaline, and nutritional supplements for the brain. Interspersed throughout the book are letters I have received from patients, testifying in their own words how these relatively simple changes brought about life-altering improvements in their health.

I have included a chapter on Fen-Phen as a point of interest because, unbeknownst to most doctors, this combination of medications had a significant effect on lowering adrenaline levels. I include also some thoughts on the "standard of care" demanded of doctors by medical review boards. Many review board experts represent the worst that medicine has to offer—if it were left to these doctors, there would be no progress in medicine, since they do not make allowances for non-traditional approaches.

If you are a patient or a healthcare practitioner who is dissatisfied with our present medical system, this book is written for you.

| CHAPTER 1 | # WHAT IS ADRENALINE DOMINANCE? |

Consider for a moment the following three cases:

Case I: A 58-year-old man who is the CEO of a software company comes to see his doctor, complaining of trouble falling asleep. He tosses and turns through the night. When he does finally fall asleep, he grinds his teeth. He is on high blood pressure medication and an antidepressant. He has a tendency to drink more alcohol than he should. When sitting, one knee often twitches up and down involuntarily. His wife tells him that during the night his legs move constantly. At work he has trouble focusing and is often forgetful. When he was in school he never opened a book until the night before an exam. Later on he developed a type A personality.

Case II: A 42-year-old woman hopes her doctor can help with the severe mood swings and anger issues she experiences 10 days out of the month. She often awakens around 2:30 or 3:00 a.m. and lies awake the rest of the night. She reports a problem with bladder pain and burning when she urinates. She gets shaky and irritable if she goes too long without eating. A stay-at-home mom, she is homeschooling her two children, who have both been diagnosed with ADHD and, at

1

the ages of 8 and 10, are still bed wetters. During her second pregnancy, she vomited the entire nine months.

Case III: A 50-year-old woman who is currently on disability complains of persistent fatigue. She awakens in the mornings with pain in her lower back and along the sides of her hips. She has occasional episodes of road rage. She is unable to lose the excess 42 pounds of weight she carries. She has persistent constipation, chronic headaches, and has been diagnosed with an anxiety/depression disorder. Her 30-year-old son has been diagnosed with bipolar disorder. She is on nine different medications, including one for diabetes.

These patients' complaints and concerns are problems doctors deal with on a daily basis. Between them, the three patients are presenting symptoms of the following conditions, some of which are considered incurable. These include:

- ADHD (attention deficit hyperactivity disorder)
- fibromyalgia
- depression/anxiety
- severe anger
- PMDD (premenstrual dysphoric disorder)
- IBS (irritable bowel syndrome)
- chronic interstitial cystitis
- alcoholism
- RLS (restless leg syndrome)
- insomnia
- hyperemesis gravidarum

Interestingly, every one of these conditions is related to an excess of a single hormone, adrenaline.

I refer to excess adrenaline, or hyperadrenalism, as "adrenaline dominance." It is in some ways comparable to "estrogen dominance," a term coined by John Lee, M.D. In estrogen dominance, signs and symptoms of excess estrogen, caused by an imbalance between estrogen and progesterone, lead to a variety of medical conditions, such as PMS, fibroids, and even cancer. (I write about estrogen dominance in my two other books: *The Miracle of Bio-Identical Hormones* and *The Platt Protocol for Hormone Balancing*.) Adrenaline dominance is similar, in that it also results in a variety of medical conditions. And progesterone seems to be the hormone that can help balance both excess adrenaline and excess estrogen.

Notably, most of the conditions that result from adrenaline dominance are ones for which modern medicine cannot identify the cause. Yet in my many years of experience working with patients, I have found that by viewing these conditions as caused by excess adrenaline and then choosing a treatment designed to target adrenaline and reduce it, a high percentage of my patients have been relieved of their symptoms and regained normal health.

Most of the conditions resulting from adrenaline dominance are ones for which modern medicine cannot identify the cause.

Adrenaline, also called epinephrine, is considered a "survival hormone." Large amounts of it are released when the body faces a threat of some kind. Adrenaline triggers the fight-or-flight response, which mobilizes the body's resources for immediate physical action. Adrenaline increases the sugar level in the blood and directs this energy-rich blood to the muscles, so they can fight harder or flee faster, and to the brain, which needs to be highly alert. At the same time, adrenaline constricts blood vessels that supply organs not needed in times of danger, such as the intestines. It also causes the pupils to dilate and speeds up the heart rate.

In nature, the fight-or-flight response is designed to last for only a certain period of time and then abruptly come to an end once the threat has passed. Consider, for instance, a cat threatened by a dog. The cat's body instantly releases adrenaline, directing the cat's blood supply, loaded with energy-providing sugar, to the cat's muscles and brain. After the cat has run to safety and calmed down, the high level of adrenaline drops to normal. The cat is once again relaxed, perhaps eating or taking a nap.

The human body is designed to operate similarly in its natural environment, which is how people lived for most of the millennia of human existence. Increased adrenaline prepared early humans to deal with the natural dangers that confronted them. After the danger passed, their adrenaline level, like that of the cat, presumably returned to normal.

Through the centuries, humans have drawn upon adrenaline to fight wars and deal with other dangers—real or imaginary. But now that we are in the twenty-first century, fewer people face life-threatening danger on a regular basis. A high level of adrenaline is obviously needed in some activities, such as the military, law enforcement, and sports. However, many people are putting out high levels of adrenaline all day long, even though they're not in situations that genuinely call for physical fight or flight.

Modern day life produces continuous low-level stressors in a way that is unique in human history. We are barraged by noise, too long a commute, family issues, getting burned out at work, getting too little sleep, financial concerns, no time to relax, worries about elderly parents who may be ill, problems with the kids, moving, a job transition, loss of a loved one, and other issues. Even though none of these stressors is life threatening, the body often responds to them by producing adrenaline. And because these stressors are often continuous, the adrenaline level stays high, resulting in adrenaline dominance and the health conditions it causes.

Excess adrenaline tends to create anger. It's easy to understand how this fundamental emotion goes hand in hand with facing danger—for example, when confronting a wild animal or an enemy combatant. Nowadays, however, this adrenaline-caused anger shows up frequently in non-life-threatening situations. Acting on this anger can precipitate a variety of problems such as road rage or the expressions of violence reported in newspapers almost as a daily occurrence. It is not unusual for people to internalize their anger, which leads to a number of the health conditions that are discussed later in this book.

CHAPTER 2 HOW ADRENALINE WORKS

To understand the effects of adrenaline dominance, we need a basic understanding of adrenaline's roles and functions in the body. Adrenaline is produced by the adrenal medulla, the interior part of the adrenal gland. It functions both as a hormone, controlling the activity of various tissues in the body, and as a neurotransmitter in the brain.

The body produces large amounts of adrenaline in two situations where survival may be an issue. One of these is when the body is under stress. This stress can be extreme and involving real danger—being mugged or running from a bear. Or the stress can be more emotional than physical—competitive sports, going on stage, giving a speech, being late for work, gambling, a first date, or undergoing a physical exam in a doctor's office. Both kinds of stress precipitate the release of adrenaline.

As we have seen, the release of adrenaline triggers the fight-or-flight response, which prepares the body for action. In particular, the heart rate and blood pressure rise, as does the sugar level in the blood. Blood flow to the brain and to the muscles increases, while blood flow to organs not essential to the fight-or-flight response, such as the gastrointestinal tract and the kidneys, is reduced.

The second situation that causes the release of adrenaline is when the brain is not getting enough fuel—that is, not enough sugar in the form of glucose, which is the primary source of energy used by the brain. In this situation, the body will produce sugar from protein through gluconeogenesis, a process mediated by adrenaline. Glycogen, stored in the liver, may also be converted into sugar through another process called glycogenolysis, which might also involve adrenaline.

I suspect that the most crucial reason for increased adrenaline is to provide needed fuel for the brain. The brain uses more sugar (glucose) than any other tissue in the body. When sugar is taken away from the brain, the brain falls asleep, a condition commonly known as hypoglycemia or, in extreme cases, narcolepsy. From a survival standpoint, the body will always ensure that the brain has enough fuel to be awake and alert, and it will raise the adrenaline level to accomplish this.

The most crucial reason for increased adrenaline is to provide needed fuel for the brain.

A perfect modern-day example of this survival connection is people who fall asleep while driving due to hypoglycemia— they can go right off the road, hit a tree, and kill themselves. Many times in the past I have slapped my face while driving, trying to keep awake. It usually took seven to ten minutes to wake up, which is a long time to wait while trying to avoid going off the road. I realize now that it was not the slapping that woke me up; rather, gluconeogenesis via adrenaline eventually raised my sugar level, and so I became more alert.

Besides initiating the body's own production of sugar,

hypoglycemia also stimulates a craving for foods high in sugar. High-sugar foods (such as candy, soda, cake, and cookies) are human made, not natural, so the body is not designed to handle them well. Consumption of foods high in sugar stimulates an outpouring of insulin, the hormone whose primary function is to regulate the sugar level in the blood. One of the ways insulin reduces blood sugar is by forcing sugar into muscle cells and fat cells.

The higher the sugar level in the blood, the more insulin is released. As the excess insulin pushes the excess sugar into the cells, it can precipitate another drop in the sugar level, which prompts another release of adrenaline—a sequence that can continue cyclically. This close relationship between adrenaline and insulin is a key factor in a number of health conditions, including hypertension, diabetes, unexplained weight gain, and the metabolic syndrome, or syndrome X.

Under the conditions for which adrenaline was originally designed, all or most of the elevated blood sugar would have been burned up during the fight-or-flight response. Insulin was only needed to take care of small levels of sugar that were left over. However, nowadays, because of continuous low-level stress, ongoing excess adrenaline, and not enough activity to use up the sugar, much of the sugar is not burned up. So insulin moves this extra sugar into fat cells, where it is turned into fat.

As an example, because people in law enforcement tend to have higher levels of adrenaline, they may be especially prone to getting caught in the adrenaline–sugar–insulin cycle. They famously have cravings for sugar (doughnuts?), the consumption of which produces a lot of insulin, with resultant hypoglycemia and possible weight gain. A 2011 study published in the *Journal of the American Medical Association* looked at sleep disorders affecting 5,000 police officers. The study found that 50 percent admitted to nodding off at frequent intervals while driving. These same officers were also more prone to uncontrollable anger and to committing safety violations. I suspect there may be similar issues among truck drivers who continuously fight sleepiness by eating Hostess Twinkies and taking NoDoz. Bus drivers, train engineers, and airline pilots may also be at risk for hypoglycemia—another public safety issue to consider.

Insulin is a hormone we cannot live without. However, I would not describe insulin as a "happy" hormone. Insulin is:

- the number one hormone that creates fat around the middle
- a major cause of elevated blood pressure
- the hormone that speeds up the aging process through a process called glycation
- very likely the primary cause of type II diabetes and most of the complications of diabetes

Stress can certainly stimulate the release of adrenaline. At the same time, increased adrenaline can make a person feel "stressed." Consequently, whether it is from adrenaline directly stimulating the release of cortisol from the adrenal cortex, or whether it is from increased stress stimulating the release of cortisol, either way, the end result is an increase in cortisol. One of cortisol's first functions is to increase the blood sugar level so the body has more fuel to deal with whatever is causing the stress. So now there are two hormones raising blood sugar.

Again, any time the sugar level rises, there is a concomitant increase in insulin to drive the sugar into cells, which can lead to hypoglycemia, which prompts the body to release adrenaline and cortisol to raise the sugar level again, in a cascade of hormones ad infinitum.

Cortisol, like adrenaline, is associated with increased fat around the waist because of its role in the cycle of sugar and insulin. It can also speed up osteoporosis—the same way the drug prednisone does. It also appears to have an adverse effect on the heart. High levels mean higher risk of coronary artery calcification as well as a higher number of plaques in the carotid arteries.

Over-production of cortisol also has an adverse effect on the thyroid. It causes T4 to convert into reverse T3, a form of thyroid the body cannot use. The hypothyroid state that results is not detectable if only the T4 level, and not the T3 level, is tested. Excess cortisol can also promote thyroid resistance at thyroid receptor sites. This adverse effect on thyroid function can also contribute to weight gain. Too much cortisol also impacts the pituitary gland, where it suppresses the production of thyroid stimulating hormone (TSH) as well as growth hormone (GH).

One of the benefits of the treatment program presented in this book is that it helps normalize the levels of not just adrenaline but also insulin and cortisol—the three major hormones associated with stress.

CHAPTER 3 | TREATING ADRENALINE DOMINANCE

The information on treating adrenaline dominance may be the most important material in this book. I am unaware of any other source in the medical literature that explains how to lower adrenaline. This chapter provides an overview of the adrenaline-reducing protocol. A later chapter, "Managing Excess Adrenaline," discusses the specifics of treatment in more detail.

Since stress can cause excess adrenaline, anything that reduces stress is obviously useful in lowering adrenaline. Well-known stress reducers include meditation, strenuous exercise, and deep breathing. Certain herbs can also reduce stress, such as theanine, ashwagandha, and rhodiola (all available in health food stores). These practices and herbs can help to block the effects of excess adrenaline, as can certain drugs, such as beta-blockers. These approaches, although beneficial, are actually no more than Band-Aids; they do not directly address the reason why the body is producing excess adrenaline.

To my way of thinking, successfully managing excess adrenaline requires treating the most common reason it occurs—a brain hungry for fuel. This is best achieved by following an appropriate meal plan, using a bio-identical hormone treatment, and possibly with nutritional supplementation that may be needed to support brain function. This combined approach usually brings about a significant drop in adrenaline within 24 hours, along with the elimination of many, if not all, of the patient's symptoms.

The persistence of some or all of the symptoms may mean that other factors are at work. Though adrenaline is a frequent cause of the medical conditions discussed in this book, it is not the only cause. For example, with fibromyalgia, which I feel is largely caused by internalized anger, the anger may or may not be related to adrenaline. People suffering from insomnia or depression may be reacting to specific situations in their lives. In this way, sometimes not seeing significant improvement from diet and hormones may help with identifying the specific life stressors that *are* the cause. And the treatment with diet, hormones, and supplements is still beneficial, optimizing the person's physical health while he or she takes the additional necessary steps for complete healing.

NUTRITIONAL APPROACH TO REDUCE EXCESS ADRENALINE

The nutritional aspect of my protocol for managing adrenaline focuses on the fact that hypoglycemia, or low sugar level in the brain, stimulates the production of adrenaline. The brain requires more sugar than any other body tissue. To supply the brain with fuel, the body will, if needed, synthesize sugar from protein through metabolic pathways that involve adrenaline.

The brain can be low in sugar for two reasons. One is the overproduction of insulin, which causes the blood sugar level to drop. The body produces the most insulin after eating and also in the midafternoon. People who get sleepy after eating or between 3 and 4 p.m. more than likely will release adrenaline at these times to counteract this drop in sugar. The second reason is that the person is not eating correctly. A key principle in eating to control adrenaline is to eat low-glycemic rather than high-glycemic carbohydrates. The glycemic index rates foods (mostly carbohydrates) according to how quickly or slowly they are digested. High-glycemic foods are digested more quickly, so sugar is released into the blood stream quickly. Low-glycemic foods are digested more slowly and release sugar more steadily. The bottom line is that high-glycemic foods stimulate the production of more insulin.

High-glycemic carbohydrates are primarily refined carbohydrates, such as white rice, white bread, sugar of all kinds, corn, bananas, and so on. They cause a quick rise in blood glucose (sugar) that stimulates the release of large amounts of insulin, which then leads to hypoglycemia and, subsequently, production of adrenaline.

Green vegetables are the perfect fuel for the brain.

Low-glycemic carbohydrates cause a smaller, slower rise in glucose in the blood and do not stimulate as much insulin release. Types of low-glycemic foods include green vegetables, certain starchy vegetables, unprocessed grains, and legumes. Among these types, green vegetables are the perfect fuel for the brain. They can be consumed in a vegetable omelet or in scrambled eggs, added to a green smoothie or a salad, or eaten as a side dish. Examples of low-glycemic foods include sweet potatoes; brown rice, brown rice pasta, brown rice tortillas, oatmeal; and pinto or black beans.

The importance of eating correctly to manage adrenaline should not be underestimated. Without the proper nutrition to keep the blood sugar level steady, people may find themselves "living on adrenaline" as the body continuously releases adrenaline in order to manufacture its own sugar so the body and brain can have sufficient fuel. People who skip breakfast or only eat once a day are probably in this category. Adrenaline also takes away the appetite. Those who put out adrenaline during the night may find they have no appetite in the morning.

The meal plan provided later in the book includes a discussion of low-glycemic carbohydrates, sample meal plans, and smoothie recipes, as well as general dietary advice. There is no one-size-fits-all approach to how people with excess adrenaline should be eating. The meal plan should be considered only as a set of guidelines, to be fine-tuned to suit each person.

HORMONAL APPROACH TO REDUCE EXCESS ADRENALINE

Only one hormone is needed to help control adrenaline: progesterone. Progesterone is applied in the form of a bio-identical transdermal cream, available by prescription from a compounding pharmacy, or it can be obtained in lower strengths without a prescription.

Progesterone provides a two-pronged approach for managing excess adrenaline: it reduces the secretion of adrenaline by preventing insulin-induced hypoglycemia, and it appears to directly block the effects of adrenaline.

I am not aware of the physiological pathways by which progesterone affects insulin, since there are no studies delineating this. I suspect it could prevent the action of insulin at insulin receptor sites, or it might possibly affect the release of insulin by the beta cells of the pancreas. However, I am convinced of its significant effect on insulin based on feedback from thousands of patients as well as my own experience using it. Patients who use progesterone correctly no longer experience hypoglycemic sleepiness caused by high insulin, most commonly noted after eating, or between 3 and 4 in the afternoon, or while traveling in a car, whether as the driver or as a passenger. In addition, they often experience weight loss.

Progesterone provides a two-pronged approach for managing excess adrenaline: it reduces the secretion of adrenaline by preventing insulin-induced hypoglycemia, and it directly blocks the effects of adrenaline.

As the episodes of hypoglycemia become fewer, the production of adrenaline to counteract hypoglycemia also drops. Less adrenaline means less sugar is produced, and thus also less insulin.

Progesterone seems to directly counteract adrenaline's effects most dramatically in patients whose level of adrenaline is especially high. Sitting in my office, they often remarked on how much better they felt less than three minutes after applying progesterone cream for the first time. Their leg tapping disappeared, they sat back in their chair, they felt more relaxed, and they were able to focus better.

Besides helping to control insulin and blocking adrenaline, progesterone has other positive effects on the body, including blocking the effects of estrogen dominance, or excess estrogen, in women. Excess estrogen can have harmful side effects— cramps, PMS, breast tenderness, and migraine headaches. Over time, estrogen dominance can lead to fibroids, endometriosis, PCOS, asthma, and gallbladder disease, and can be the cause of six different cancers in women, especially breast cancer. All women on birth control pills are estrogen dominant because the pill prevents ovulation, so they no longer produce progesterone. Morning sickness during a woman's first trimester is another effect of estrogen dominance.

A number of factors should be taken into consideration with regard to prescribing transdermal bio-identical progesterone cream:

1. There is no one-size-fits-all dosage for progesterone. Rather, the patient begins with a generally recommended dosage and then adapts the amount, frequency of application, and even application site as needed.

2. When it comes to dosing progesterone, it is better to treat the patient rather than a lab test—that is, adjust the dosage according to the patient's response rather than blood test results.

3. It is best applied to areas with a good blood supply where the skin is thin— for example, the inner forearm, the upper chest, the back of the neck, or the face.

4. It appears to be extremely safe with few potential side effects.

5. Progesterone has a short half-life in the blood stream (about five to six minutes) because of its propensity to attach readily to receptor sites.

6. Bio-identical progesterone is not the same as a progestin such as Provera, which is not bio-identical and has the same side effects as estrogen, including cancer. In contrast, bio-identical progesterone appears to prevent every cancer that estrogen causes.

7. Saliva tests do not give an accurate picture of progesterone levels, except perhaps in people not using the transdermal cream.

8. Oral progesterone, which comes in capsules or troches, should be avoided. It goes straight to the liver, where it converts primarily into a different hormone called allopregnanolone. This hormone causes drowsiness, which is why oral progesterone is given at night.

SUPPLEMENTS FOR THE BRAIN

Most people with excess adrenaline complain of having difficulty focusing their attention. This may be caused by excess adrenaline in the brain speeding up thought processes. When the brain is working faster, some of the biochemical nutrients it needs in order to function may get depleted—just as increased muscle function, caused by adrenaline, will consume various nutrients utilized by the muscles.

In addition, adrenaline as a neurotransmitter in the brain interacts with other neurotransmitters. When adrenaline levels are elevated, the other neurotransmitters must be affected too, influencing how we think and feel.

People who have had a lifetime of excess adrenaline may sustain damage to certain brain cells. In this regard, excess adrenaline can produce stress, which can lead to an increase in the production of cortisol. Prolonged stress associated with this increase in cortisol leads to damage of the hippocampus, a part of the brain that has many receptors for cortisol. The hippocampus is involved in cognition, mood, and memory. Over time, the damage can cause memory problems, dementia, and depression.

Fortunately, the body has an amazing capacity to heal itself. In the old days, eating a healthy diet was enough to provide all the necessary elements needed for healthy brain function. Unfortunately, it is a different world today. Because of pollution, depletion of the soil, and the use of chemical fertilizers and now GMO seeds, the nutritional quality of our food is less than it was one hundred years ago. As a result, for optimal health we require the support of nutritional supplements, including for the brain.

While the topic of proper metabolic support for brain cells is too complex to discuss in detail in this book, the most important supplements for the brain are listed and discussed in the chapter "Managing Excess Adrenaline."

CHAPTER 4 | EXCESS ADRENALINE: THE GOOD

To my way of thinking, ADHD (attention deficit hyperactivity disorder) is all about excess adrenaline. I regard it as the "good" aspect of adrenaline dominance because, when managed properly, the tendency toward elevated adrenaline leads to heightened cognition, creativity, and capacity to get things done. Many of the world's most intelligent, successful, creative people have been diagnosed as having ADHD or have exhibited many of ADHD's symptoms.

ADHD represents a classic example of the tendency to judge a condition by its symptoms rather than by its cause. As a result, children with ADHD are described as having a learning disorder, or having trouble focusing, or being prone to disruptive behaviors or temper tantrums, and so on.

All of these symptoms are related to adrenaline. As a hormone, excess adrenaline increases energy to muscles, leading to hyperactivity. As a neurotransmitter, it can heighten awareness and intelligence. However, it also increases the speed of thought transmission, making it difficult to focus, except on subjects that are of interest. If the subject on the blackboard is not interesting, a child with ADHD can get easily distracted—looking out the window, talking to the child at the next desk, and so on. However, put the same child in front of a computer with games, and he or she might be able to focus on it for the better part of a day.

In other words, ADHD is not actually a learning disorder; it's an interest disorder. A classic example of ADHD is the student with excellent grades in all subjects except, say, algebra. This is clearly an intelligent student who finds it difficult to focus on a certain subject.

In my view, there are three basic forms of ADHD, which I call "typical type," "creative type," and "mixed type," the last being a combination of the first two types. In typical type ADHD, adrenaline functions primarily as a hormone, acting on the muscles to cause physical hyperactivity and possibly impulsive or even disruptive behavior. In creative type ADHD, adrenaline functions mainly as a neurotransmitter in the brain, making the brain hyperactive. This form of ADHD is more common in people who are "right brained," that is, creative. The adrenaline enhances their creativity.

In typical type ADHD, adrenaline functions primarily as a hormone. In creative type ADHD, adrenaline functions mainly as a neurotransmitter in the brain.

I suspect that most people diagnosed as having ADD (attention deficit disorder) actually have what I call creative type ADHD. The difference in the name is crucial, since retaining the "H" in "ADHD" identifies this condition as a form of hyperactivity, though in this case the hyperactivity is in the brain. These people have trouble focusing, similar to those with what is generally called ADHD, but they lack the physical hyperactivity and impulsiveness. Understanding that this condition is another form of adrenaline hyperactivity is vital to treating it properly.

The latest estimate of ADHD in children (2013) is 10 percent, though I believe that the true incidence is much higher. If the negative connotations of this disorder were removed, I suspect that a lot more children might be diagnosed and correctly treated.

In addition, if one parent has ADHD, there is a good chance of the children having ADHD. If both parents have ADHD, then all of their children will have ADHD. Conversely, if a child has ADHD, it is a good bet that one or both parents have it as well.

It is important to keep in mind that all children with ADHD grow up to be adults with ADHD. The condition does not magically disappear at the age of 18.

It should not be surprising that ADHD in most adults goes unrecognized by the medical community. It should also not be surprising that the medical community considers many conditions associated with adult ADHD—the "bad" and "ugly" aspects of excess adrenaline—incurable. We are dealing here with hormones out of balance, a concept that is not recognized by many physicians.

As a neurotransmitter in the brain, adrenaline helps to increase intelligence; as a hormone, it enhances physical energy. This combination of energy and mental acumen produces the most successful people in the world. Many successful people today will admit that they never opened a book in school until the night before an exam. They may have been branded as procrastinators, but they did well scholastically anyway because of their brain's hyperactivity. In my own case, I never studied until the night before an exam. However, when I got into medical school I studied at least three or four hours every night because I was interested in medicine.

Most people whose work requires thinking skills, such as lawyers, doctors, and scientists, as well as the heads of almost every corporation, by my definition probably have ADHD. For example, Bill Gates, as most people are aware, left college after his second year, obviously not because of lack of intelligence. People have observed that he paces a lot, rocks back and forth in his chair, and taps his foot all the time. These are all symptoms of too much adrenaline.

TYPICAL TYPE ADHD

People with what I call typical type ADHD are inclined to be physically active. They are intelligent but may have trouble focusing. As adults, they might smoke too much or drink too much. Sometimes they have anxiety issues. They often have a history of being easily irritated and quick to anger, even road rage, and may have high expectations of other people.

As children they may be thin, since their hyperactivity allows them to burn up sugar before it can be stored as fat. As they approach middle age, they are less active and may start putting on weight around the middle, caused by excess insulin. The excess insulin can also cause symptoms of hypoglycemia: sleepiness in the late afternoon or after eating or while traveling in a car.

People with typical type ADHD commonly display other symptoms of high adrenaline. These include restlessness—tapping their hands or feet during the day, restless leg syndrome, tossing and turning or grinding their teeth at night—and they may have trouble falling asleep. Stated another way, adrenaline can be considered a form of natural speed.

People with typical type ADHD are inclined to be physically active and display other symptoms of high adrenaline, such as restlessness and having trouble falling asleep.

There is frequently a strong family history of associated hormonal problems—a brother who is bipolar, children or nephews and nieces who are hyperactive, relatives who have type II diabetes or fibromyalgia. Since ADHD is associated with low progesterone levels among the women in the family, there may be a history of breast cancer, endometriosis, or other conditions associated with estrogen dominance.

Characteristically, when hyperactive children get into high school and college, they often get involved in sports, and later on in life they often become type A personalities or workaholics. Adrenaline drives high activity. It is the hormone that allows people in certain professions to perform their jobs. Men and women involved in the military, law enforcement, or professional sports can attribute many of their abilities to adrenaline. I suspect that many of these people had the classic symptoms of typical type ADHD when they were younger.

Children with typical type ADHD are often treated with drugs such as Ritalin, Adderall, or Strattera, which actually increase the level of adrenaline in the brain. Because they increase adrenaline, these drugs can have the effect of numbing the brain. They can also cause serious side effects, including sudden death or suicide. On the other hand, treating this condition with progesterone, diet, and nutritional supplements can, in most cases, eliminate many of the unwanted symptoms of ADHD without the need for medications.

Although I generally have not seen children as patients in my practice, I have occasionally treated them in the course of treating their parents. One nine-year-old boy, Jose, who had a classic case of typical type ADHD, had been thrown out of every public school in his hometown for aggressive behavior, including fighting with other children and shoving teachers. His mother, who was my patient, was desperate because the boy sincerely wanted to go back to school. So I agreed to meet with him.

In the course of the appointment, I learned that Jose was addicted to sugar; everything he ate and drank was sugar-based. I sat down with him and explained that in order to get better and be able to go back to school, his diet had to change. I told him he would be putting a cream on his lower forearm. He agreed and was given a meal plan to follow.

Twenty-four hours later, his mother called me and told me she could not stop crying; she had never seen her son behave so well. He had just completed ten pages of homework—quite an accomplishment for someone who had never done homework before. His symptoms of excess adrenaline were gone.

In spite of his recovery, the school board refused to readmit him. I wrote a two-page letter of explanation, but the public educational system was blind to his condition. Eventually he enrolled in a parochial school, where he became first in his class after six months. This is not surprising, since most ADHD children are extremely intelligent.

The psychiatrist who had been following Jose for his ADHD noticed right away that the signs of this disorder were gone. When he asked Jose's mother what her son was using and she said progesterone cream, he told her to stop the cream immediately, that it was a female hormone. He said she should put him back on the drugs previously prescribed. She explained that Jose wouldn't take them because they made him feel sick. He told her to do it anyway. Needless to say, the mother let Jose continue with the cream.

I subsequently spoke with the psychiatrist, who refused to accept what I was saying because it was unverifiable by drug company studies. His statement that progesterone is a female hormone typifies many doctors' lack of education about hormones. Progesterone is present in men just as it is present in women. This physician refused to rely on his own powers of observation and acknowledge that progesterone was beneficial. He would rather place this nine-year-old boy on potentially lethal drugs, with multiple side effects, than use a natural bio-identical hormone with no side effects.

CREATIVE TYPE ADHD

While people with typical type ADHD are highly intelligent and highly active, those with what I call creative type ADHD have high intelligence along with heightened creativity.

Research has shown that the left hemisphere of the brain is responsible mainly for logical, rational thinking, while the right hemisphere is primarily responsible for creative, intuitive, and feelings-based thinking. A right-brained person who has a lot of adrenaline in the brain as a neurotransmitter can be a creative genius. My personal opinion is that highly creative thinkers like Albert Einstein, Beethoven, Shakespeare, and Leonardo da Vinci all had creative type ADHD.

Because mental hyperactivity is generally not as noticeable as physical hyperactivity, the fact that it is a form of ADHD can go unnoticed. However, it is especially important to recognize the creative type ADHD person. The creative brain requires a lot more sugar than a normal brain because it is more active.

If these people are not treated correctly, they will continuously be pouring out adrenaline to raise the brain's sugar level—a situation resulting in some of the dire conditions discussed in the chapters that follow.

Because mental hyperactivity is not as noticeable as physical hyperactivity, the fact that it is a form of ADHD can go unnoticed. However, it is especially important to recognize the creative type ADHD person.

Those with creative type ADHD are likely to also have symptoms caused by adrenaline acting as a hormone. Characteristically, if they go too long without eating, they get shaky or irritable, which is caused by the release of adrenaline to raise the sugar level. They may experience cold hands and feet due to constriction of blood vessels. An extremely common problem is weight gain. At night, they usually have trouble staying asleep. This is because the brain, which continues to work even during sleep, can run out of fuel around 2:30 or 3:00 a.m., which is the classic time that adrenaline is released to raise sugar levels. This in turn causes them to awaken. Increased adrenaline during the night often results in the mind racing, generalized restlessness, grinding of the teeth or TMJ, low back or hip pain due to muscle tension, or waking up to urinate during the night.

Through the years I have noted certain reliable characteristics of people who have creative type ADHD. For example, they are often intuitive about others, that is, they can pick up good or bad "vibes." It is not unusual for them to have premonitions or experiences of déjà vu. They may know who's on the phone before they answer it, or they answer by saying, "I was just thinking of you," or "I was getting ready to call you." Animals are attracted to them, as are babies and small children. Clairvoyants and psychics are often people with creative type ADHD, as are horse whisperers, dog whisperers, and baby whisperers (the nurses who can quiet crying babies just by holding them). Creative type ADHD patients of mine who live in rural areas have reported birds landing next to them or on their arm, or deer coming up to them and eating out of their hand.

My own conjecture about these phenomena is that somehow the energy created by adrenaline in a right-side-dominant brain is able to tap into the energies in the air, such as those caused by cell phone, WiFi, and satellite transmissions. Small children who are themselves creative, as well as animals, can sense this energy in creative people and are attracted to it.

A classic symptom of people with creative type ADHD is the tendency to fall asleep while traveling in a car, especially as a passenger. This may be due to the large amount of sensory input coming into the brain, which is registering all the passing scenery as well as other cars on the road, while also listening to the radio, talking to the driver, and so on. As a result, the brain runs out of fuel and the person falls asleep.

I suspect that people who make their living in creative careers—artists, dancers, musicians, graphic designers, creative chefs, interior designers, writers, beauticians, people with an uncanny ability to fix motors, architects, and innovators in all fields—are likely to have creative type ADHD. In this regard, movie stars deserve special mention. It is not unusual for events involving them to make the newswires—the rages of Mel Gibson, Alec Baldwin, Michael Richards; the drug problems of Lindsay Lohan, Heath Ledger, Charlie Sheen,

Robert Downey Jr., and Whitney Houston. I believe all these situations are related to excess adrenaline. A tragedy that occurred in Los Angeles exemplifies how powerful adrenaline can be. A man was making his way across the street in a marked crosswalk. An approaching car pulled to a stop somewhat over the line, with its front protruding into the crosswalk space. The pedestrian went into what I would call "crosswalk rage" and pounded the hood of the car as he walked by. The driver of the car had "road rage"—he got out of the car, pushed the other fellow down to the ground, and kicked him repeatedly in the head, killing him. Just to make sure, he got back in his car and drove over the body.

It turned out that both men were musicians, that is, creative people, very likely with creative type ADHD. Based on how easily each of them went into a rage, I would guess that both men were living on adrenaline (relying primarily on adrenaline to provide fuel for the brain). If just one of them had been diagnosed and treated correctly, this tragedy could have been avoided.

Perhaps the classic example of the power of adrenaline in a creative person is Michael Jackson. The following is my evaluation of what caused his death, based on information generally available. At his death, this extremely creative man was emaciated. His highly creative brain required large amounts of sugar for fuel, but high adrenaline took away his appetite, which would explain his extreme weight loss. It also explains why he couldn't sleep at night and required huge amounts of ineffectual, toxic sleeping aids.

He maintained this poor state of health until he signed a contract to perform 50 concerts in London beginning the summer of 2009. In preparation, he started rehearsing at the

Staples Center in Los Angeles. For the first time in about ten years he was up on stage going through his dance routines. This meant that his muscles needed extra fuel to burn. Since he still wasn't getting an adequate amount of nutrition, his body now had to produce even more adrenaline to raise his sugar level, which created even more sleeping problems. Eventually, the excess adrenaline may have stopped his heart—just three weeks before the concerts were to begin. The medications he was receiving might have contributed, as well.

MIXED TYPE ADHD

Some people manifest characteristics of both types of ADHD, a condition I call mixed type ADHD. They seem to have excess adrenaline in the brain plus increased adrenaline as a systemic hormone. In my experience, people with mixed ADHD have more severe symptoms than people with either the typical or the creative type. They have more problems with anxiety, obsessive-compulsive behaviors, or depression, and sometimes have the most difficulty focusing. Women with this condition may have increased nausea throughout an entire pregnancy.

These are the people who may have been diagnosed as having dyslexia—the tendency to read letters or numbers backwards. They are both right-brained and left-brained. Often enough, they may also be the most successful people in the world.

THOUGHTS ON ADHD AND ADRENALINE

To summarize, I feel that ADHD represents the good side of excess adrenaline. People whose work requires brainpower can often thank their high level of adrenaline for their intelligence. Professional athletes can attribute much of their skill and strength to adrenaline. People in law enforcement and in the military rely on adrenaline to do their work. However, unless properly treated, people with ADHD are likely to also experience the down sides of adrenaline, which are discussed in the following chapters.

From my experience with thousands of patients, I can say that treating ADHD associated with excess adrenaline with the proper meal plan and progesterone therapy addresses the problem directly and surprisingly quickly. Yet the link between ADHD and adrenaline is not yet generally recognized. In the last year alone, more than a thousand articles on ADHD were published in medical journals. Not one of them mentioned adrenaline.

This is certain to change, eventually. I predict that about 20 years from now someone will receive the Nobel Prize in Medicine for figuring out the cause of ADHD and ADD. It may take that long for the medical establishment to appreciate the fact that a hormone imbalance involving excess adrenaline is the root cause.

CHAPTER 5 | EXCESS ADRENALINE: THE BAD

All of the conditions included in the three excess adrenaline categories—the "good," the "bad," and the "ugly"—affect the quality of life of the people who have them. The ones I have placed in the "bad" category, in my view, may not impact the patient as severely as those in the "ugly" category. However, the distinction between "bad" and "ugly" is somewhat arbitrary. In fact, the same person can have symptoms relevant to all three categories.

The majority of the conditions caused by excessive amounts of adrenaline, an extremely powerful hormone, are considered incurable. Standard medical practice for these conditions is to prescribe medications that often have adverse effects on the body while failing to provide much relief; this is because the medications primarily alleviate the conditions' symptoms, not their cause. I have seen this repeatedly in patients who have come to my office in desperation, their bodies burdened with the effects of both excess adrenaline and their medications. The speed and magnitude of their relief when they begin a treatment that targets excess adrenaline, along with weaning themselves off the drugs, is rewarding to both patient and practitioner.

It is my feeling that doctors are at a crossroads. They can continue their present course of practice, which means accepting the fact that their patients will rarely get better, or they can challenge the status quo, remember the Hippocratic Oath they took when getting their degree, and practice a kind of medicine their patients will appreciate. The Oath says, in part: "I will apply, for the benefit of the sick, all measures that are required, avoiding those twin traps of overtreatment and therapeutic nihilism." This and other excerpts from the Oath are included in the chapter "Standard of Care." "Therapeutic nihilism" refers to ignoring moral principles when practicing medicine. For current examples we need look no further than the 100,000 people who die from prescription drugs and the 400,000 people who wind up hospitalized because of drug reactions every year. In my experience, patients, if given the choice, have almost always elected to eliminate the underlying cause of a problem rather than take a medication that can cause unpleasant or even disastrous side effects.

It is my feeling that doctors are at a crossroads. They can continue their present course of practice, or they can challenge the status quo.

In this and the next chapter my intention is not to explore all the characteristics and ramifications of the diseases discussed. Rather, I explain the basics of each condition and how it is an effect of excess adrenaline. All of these discussions, assessments, and recommendations are based on my experience working with and gathering feedback from thousands of patients over several decades.

DEPRESSION

Depression is a fairly common mood disorder that affects most people at one time or another. Characterized by loss of interest or feeling sad or helpless, it may have other associated symptoms, such as trouble sleeping, aches and pains, and loss of appetite.

Clinically significant depression affects 5 to 10 percent of the population. To make this diagnosis, five of the following nine major criteria, listed in the *Diagnostic and Statistical Manual of Mental Disorders (DSM-IV)* must be present nearly every day:

1. Depressed mood or irritability
2. Loss of interest or pleasure
3. Significant weight loss or gain
4. Insomnia or hypersomnia
5. Psychomotor agitation or retardation
6. Fatigue or loss of energy
7. Feelings of worthlessness, or excessive or inappropriate guilt
8. Diminished ability to think or concentrate or make decisions
9. Recurrent thoughts of death or suicide

There are basically two types of depression: reactive and endogenous. Reactive depression is related to some negative event in the person's life, such as loss of a job, financial problems, or loss of a loved one (including a pet). Endogenous depression comes from within—the person is depressed but doesn't know why. A third type of depression can manifest as a combination of reactive and endogenous.

I believe that excess adrenaline is the number one cause of endogenous depression. How is this so? I have observed that a high adrenaline level is the most common cause of anger problems. Anger is a very powerful emotion. While some people let it out in various ways—hitting a wall, yelling, fighting, etc.—others hold it inside. A tremendous amount of negative energy can build up within them, even if they don't realize it. When anger is unconsciously suppressed, it can show up as depression.

Except in rare cases, I have been able to help hundreds of patients successfully get rid of their depression as well as wean themselves off their antidepressant medications just by lowering their adrenaline levels.

ANXIETY

Anxiety disorder is the most common mental illness in the United States, affecting over 40 million adults, or about 20 percent of the U.S. population. Anxiety is frequently associated with a depressive disorder—people who are depressed are nearly nine times more likely to develop an anxiety disorder than people who are not.

The criteria in the *DSM-IV* for generalized anxiety disorder include:

1. At least six months of excessive anxiety or worry

2. Significant difficulty in controlling the anxiety or worry

3. For six months, the presence of three or more of the following symptoms on most days:

   - Feeling wound up, tense, or restless

   - Becoming easily fatigued or worn out

- Concentration problems
- Irritability
- Significant tension in muscles
- Difficulty with sleep

It is easy to see how adrenaline can be responsible for a number of symptoms of this disorder: restlessness, fatigue caused by prolonged muscle tension, insomnia, nervousness, and jitteriness. People struggling with anxiety often feel the need to smoke or drink or take drugs to relax. It is not unusual for them to crave sugary foods.

Adrenaline can be responsible for a number of anxiety symptoms: restlessness, fatigue caused by prolonged muscle tension, insomnia, nervousness, and jitteriness.

Generalized anxiety disorder is a medical condition characterized by fear, unease, and worry while not being able to identify the source of these feelings. There are other types of anxiety disorders, including panic disorder (acute anxiety reaction), obsessive-compulsive disorder, and post-traumatic stress disorder (PTSD). I discuss PTSD briefly in the next chapter.

Panic disorder, a disabling condition associated with anxiety, affects about 6 million people in the United States. It is characterized by sudden and repeated attacks of intense fear, known as panic attacks, which occur when there is no real danger. The classic symptoms are:

- Shortness of breath (air hunger)
- Palpitations
- A sense of impending doom

Because of the feeling of air hunger, or shortness of breath, the person hyperventilates, expelling too much carbon dioxide. Hyperventilation can result in pain on the left side of the chest secondary to gas pain from swallowed air. It can also cause numbness and tingling around the lips and fingers as the blood becomes more alkaline from blowing off carbon dioxide.

A patient suffering from a panic attack may show up at the emergency room complaining of chest pain and shortness of breath—classic symptoms of a possible heart attack. This, of course, gives the hospital a reason to do an expensive workup, even though a panic attack, or acute anxiety attack, is one of the easiest diagnoses in medicine to make, as shown in the movie *Something's Gotta Give*. The character played by Jack Nicholson comes to the emergency room complaining of shortness of breath and chest pain. However, after his EKG and cardiac enzymes test normal, the emergency room doctor reassures him that he is having an anxiety reaction. In real life, many more expensive though unnecessary tests might be run as well, such as an echocardiogram, a thallium stress test, and possibly an angiogram, even though they might not be necessary.

People with anxiety issues often have sighing-type respirations. They may have the sensation of a lump in their throat, referred to as globus hystericus, caused by muscle contraction in that area.

If reducing adrenaline does not completely eliminate a person's panic attacks, he or she may be dealing with suppressed hostility or resentment. These feelings are often deep in the subconscious, where the person is not aware of them. When the suppressed hostility starts coming into the conscious mind, it can result in a panic attack, which is the body's attempt to push the hostility back into the subconscious. This suppressed hostility is usually toward somebody close to the person. In these cases, the person needs to look back over his or her life and see if a parent or sibling or spouse or even a child has been the cause of an emotional hurt. The treatment is to deal directly with the issue that has been suppressed.

Obsessive-compulsive behavior, another anxiety-related problem, can take the form of ritualized behaviors, such as obsessive hand washing, or repeatedly checking to see if doors are locked or lights have been turned off. This type of behavior is actually a defense mechanism to keep the person from experiencing anxiety. In other words, if a person with a need to perform an obsessive act is prevented from doing so, he or she will experience anxiety. Again, lowering the adrenaline level often helps to eliminate the need to perform obsessive acts.

IRRITABLE BOWEL SYNDROME

Irritable bowel syndrome, or IBS—also called spastic colitis—is characterized by constipation, diarrhea, or some combination of both, although the most common manifestation of this disorder is constipation. During the fight-or-flight response, caused by the release of adrenaline, extra blood is sent to the muscles while circulation to the internal organs, which includes the intestines, is reduced. This can result in a slowdown of intestinal motility.

Constipation is one of the most common gastrointestinal expressions of excess adrenaline. In addition, when powerful feelings caused by adrenaline, such as anger and irritability, are internalized, they can result in diarrhea or intestinal spasms.

Disorders associated with diarrhea are separated into two categories: organic and functional. Organic diarrhea occurs both day and night. Examples include ulcerative colitis, regional enteritis (Crohn's disease), ischemic colitis, and diarrhea caused by the bacteria *C. difficile* or by the protozoa *Giardia lamblia*, which causes giardiasis. Functional diarrheas are regarded as psychological in origin and are not usually associated with having to get up at night with diarrhea. Irritable bowel syndrome is in this category.

I have observed that other chronic inflammatory bowel conditions, such as ulcerative colitis and regional enteritis (Crohn's disease), are similarly exacerbated by internalizing anger. Very often this anger is related to relationships with family members. Reducing the person's adrenaline level often significantly improves his or her interactions with others, along with a significant improvement in gastrointestinal symptoms.

HYPERTENSION

I suspect that many cases of hypertension are related to excess adrenaline. As part of the fight-or-flight response, adrenaline can certainly raise blood pressure. "White coat hypertension," a classic condition in which a person's blood pressure rises while it is being measured in a doctor's office, is caused by the release of adrenaline. Since visiting a doctor's office is not the only source of stress in this world, a person who has white coat hypertension most likely has frequent episodes of hypertension in other life situations.

Similarly, it is not unusual for blood pressure to spike in a dental office secondary to receiving a shot of novocaine mixed with epinephrine. In this case, epinephrine (which is adrenaline) is used to control bleeding because it causes blood vessels to constrict. Admittedly, the mere sight of a dental drill can induce fear in many people, with a concomitant rise in adrenaline that leads to a spike in blood pressure.

If adrenaline is rising, then so is blood sugar. Any time the blood sugar level goes up, the body produces insulin to move the sugar into the cells where it is needed. Insulin is also a hormone that raises blood pressure, a fact well demonstrated by the condition called metabolic syndrome, or syndrome X. This condition is indicated by high triglycerides, low HDL cholesterol, and a high insulin level, as well as hypertension. To my knowledge, the only cause of a low HDL is elevated insulin.

In addition, excess adrenaline is associated with increased stress. When under stress, the body releases cortisol, another hormone that stimulates sugar production, which leads to more insulin production, which can further increase blood pressure. The excess insulin can also cause a drop in blood sugar (hypoglycemia), which stimulates the production of adrenaline to increase sugar, which again raises blood pressure as well as cortisol, ad infinitum. This scenario of cascading hormones is likely to cause recurrent and/or persistent hypertension.

Wouldn't it make more sense to just lower adrenaline and avoid using drugs that can cause impotence, weight gain, bronchial spasm leading to asthma, plus other side effects?

The proximal cause of all the aforementioned scenarios is excess adrenaline. Elevated blood pressure is commonly treated with a beta-blocker, such as atenolol, metoprolol, or propranalol, which blocks the effects of adrenaline. Wouldn't it make more sense to just lower adrenaline and avoid using a class of drugs that can cause impotence, weight gain (they are antithyroid drugs), bronchial spasm leading to asthma, plus other side effects? High adrenaline can be easily controlled with diet and hormones, and then the patient can gradually wean himself or herself off the antihypertensive medications.

DIABETES

The two most common types of diabetes are type I and type II. Type I diabetes is caused by lack of insulin. Type II (adult onset) diabetes is commonly thought to be caused by *resistance* to insulin—that is, the cells become resistant to the action of insulin, so sugar has difficulty getting into the cells. However, I, along with a small but growing number of physicians, feel that type II diabetes is actually caused by the *overproduction* of insulin.

A growing number of physicians feel that type II diabetes is actually caused by the *overproduction* of insulin.

This view of type II diabetes is controversial and contrary to the traditional approach. However, the traditional approach is clearly not working. Attempts to lower blood sugar levels with drugs that increase insulin production or with insulin itself, as well as to lower cholesterol levels and blood pressure, usually all fail to prevent the complications of diabetes. In fact, those studies that have attempted to reduce sugar levels to normal in diabetics by increasing insulin to a high level have resulted in an alarming increase in mortality and complications. In 2012, the normal level for hemoglobin A1C, the time-honored measurement of diabetic control, was raised from 6.5 to 7.5, an indication that diabetes experts may be realizing that lowering sugar levels by increasing insulin is not the answer. Standard thinking about diabetes is that sugar cannot get into the cells because all the cells are resistant to insulin; therefore the sugar stays in the bloodstream. However, I have suspected for some time that an additional factor might be involved: that the sugar cannot be transported into fat cells for storage purposes because the fat cells have become saturated with fat (i.e., there is no more room at the inn). As a result, the sugar level in the blood goes up.

The importance of dealing with insulin in type II diabetes cannot be overstated. Insulin is a fat-storing hormone. It creates fat by pushing sugar into fat cells, where it is converted into fat for storage; it also sits outside fat cells and blocks the release of fat. Insulin is recognized as the cause of fat accumulating around the abdomen. People who produce a lot of insulin often have a paunch around the middle and relatively thin legs and arms. I suspect that when the fat cells in the abdominal area fill up, diabetes can follow.

Let's look at this more closely. The number of fat cells we have throughout life is generally determined at a very young age. People who were thin early in life often have fewer fat cells as adults. Because they have fewer fat cells to absorb sugar, they may be predisposed to developing adult-onset diabetes. (I have observed that some women who have undergone significant liposuction procedures can develop a type of diabetes that is often incurable—they have run out of fat cells in which to store sugar.) The current epidemic of type II diabetes among teenagers might very well be due to a combination of how they eat, lack of exercise to burn off sugar, excessive adrenaline (which raises both sugar and insulin), and, in some cases, having been thin early in life.

If type II diabetes is caused by excess insulin, where does the excess insulin come from? In my view, adrenaline is the root cause. Overproduction of adrenaline leads to overproduction of sugar in order to fuel the brain and muscles. The elevated blood sugar stimulates the release of insulin.

At the same time, overproduction of adrenaline also causes the release of cortisol. Cortisol, like adrenaline, raises the blood sugar level, which stimulates the release of insulin.

As we have seen, elevated insulin lowers blood sugar (hypoglycemia). And low blood sugar stimulates cravings for food high in sugar as well as the release of more adrenaline (and cortisol), and so the cycle continues.

This cycle can also include the release of glucagon, another hormone that can raise the sugar level. So now three hormones are raising the sugar level, which is further exacerbated if the person eats foods high in sugar. Is it any wonder that people wind up with high sugar levels leading to a diagnosis of diabetes? Along the same lines, could the release of adrenaline at night be the reason that fasting sugars in the morning are often the highest sugars of the day in a diabetic?

My approach to treating type II diabetes is the same as for other medical conditions: I try to treat the underlying cause. When the insulin level is controlled, fat production is decreased and the ability to burn fat increases, so the oversaturated fat cells let go of some of their fat. Once the amount of fat inside the fat cells is reduced, there is room in those cells for sugar to get inside so the blood sugar level drops.

Compare this approach to the traditional method of treating type II diabetes. Patients are placed on medications that increase insulin production or are placed on insulin itself. In my view, these patients are being treated with the very hormone that causes not only diabetes but also most of the complications of diabetes. Not surprisingly, these patients gain more fat around the middle. They often feel sleepy between three and four in the afternoon or after eating—a sign that they are likely producing a significant amount of insulin. When a type II diabetic is taken off insulin medication in conjunction with adopting an insulin-reducing meal plan and using progesterone cream, it is not unusual for the numbness in their feet (diabetic neuropathy) to improve.

Patients on medications that increase insulin production or on insulin itself are being treated with the very hormone that causes diabetes.

To summarize my view of insulin: it contributes to accumulation of fat around the middle, it causes type II diabetes and many of the complications of diabetes, and it raises blood pressure and speeds up the aging process. Yet this is the hormone that we use to treat type II diabetics. Could this be the reason they rarely get well?

The effectiveness of reducing insulin in order to eliminate diabetes is illustrated in the following letter from a patient:

September 7, 2010
Patient J.K.
I am a retired physicist and aerospace scientist, age 82, and a patient of Dr. Platt's. In 1985, I was diagnosed with type II diabetes by my internist. The diagnosis was by glucose challenge; I had no symptoms that I recognized or complained of. I sought the best medical help I could find during subsequent years. Endocrinologists in Santa Ana, CA, UCLA Medical Center, Loma Linda Medical Center, and UCSD Medical Center treated me. I was treated with sulfonylureas, metformin, insulin, Rezulin, Avandia, and Actos. When first diagnosed, I weighed approximately 180 lbs. When I first visited Dr. Platt, January 19, 2010, I weighed 265 lbs. All of the physicians I visited suggested I lose weight, but none told me that excess insulin causes fat storage and weight gain, or that excess insulin is a characteristic of type II diabetes and of their treatment. They all encouraged me to control blood sugar. None mentioned that there is no scientific evidence that control of blood sugars to near normal levels will control diabetic complications.

Since seeing Dr. Platt in January 2010, I have understood the need to control insulin, and so I stopped all my diabetic medications. I now weigh 210 lbs., a loss of 55 lbs. I feel good. I have no retinopathy. My blood sugars are back to normal.

As I mentioned in chapter 3, I suspect that progesterone may help to control insulin by preventing the action of insulin at insulin receptor sites, which is actually a form of insulin resistance. Because insulin resistance might be a factor with certain diabetics, I recommend that they continue with metformin if they are on it, since it helps with insulin resistance. Diabetics who have creative ADHD may need to take metformin to help prevent progesterone-induced insulin resistance in brain cells.

WEIGHT PROBLEMS

When it comes to weight, the effect of adrenaline can go in either direction. On the one hand, adrenaline can increase metabolism and energy levels, which promotes the burning of fat. We often see this in children diagnosed with typical type ADHD: they are hyperactive and usually on the thin side, and in high school and college, they often participate in sports. Professional athletes are likely to have excess adrenaline, as are people designated as workaholics and type A personalities. These groups generally do not have weight issues.

On the other hand, people with excess adrenaline who are not particularly active—that is, those with creative type ADHD—may experience increased weight or be constantly fighting to prevent weight increase. The creative brain requires much more sugar than a normal brain. If the person is not eating correctly, the body will continuously put out adrenaline to raise the sugar level to supply fuel to the brain. As you might realize by now, the increase in sugar causes an increase in insulin, which pushes sugar into fat cells, where the sugar is converted into fat.

People who put out a lot of adrenaline at night are often in the unique position of gaining weight even while they are sleeping. This is in addition to the other characteristics of elevated nighttime adrenaline, such as tossing and turning, grinding teeth, restless leg syndrome, and getting up to urinate.

People who put out a lot of adrenaline at night are often in the unique position of gaining weight even while they are sleeping.

I suspect there is an unrecognized epidemic of ADHD—in particular, creative type ADHD—in which excess adrenaline is significantly raising the incidence of obesity in people of all ages. Addressing these people's weight issues from the standpoint of adrenaline could not only improve their weight but also help them to focus better.

Not only does excess adrenaline by itself contribute to weight gain, it also stimulates the release of cortisol and possibly also glucagon. So now there are two or three hormones raising the sugar level, stimulating insulin release, and creating fat.

On the other hand, excess adrenaline can also reduce a person's appetite. This is often what's happening with people who regularly skip breakfast: they release so much adrenaline during the night that they don't want to eat in the morning. They can end up essentially living on adrenaline through the persistent cyclical release of sugar and insulin it precipitates. Excess adrenaline can also create a craving to drink alcohol in order to relax—another potential cause of weight gain.

In addition, medications prescribed for medical conditions caused by excess adrenaline can encourage increased weight. Both the antidepressants given to people with anger issues or depression and the beta-blockers frequently prescribed for people with hypertension or palpitations can cause weight gain. The drugs that type II diabetics are frequently given to raise the insulin level also create fat.

I would be remiss if I did not also mention how our healthcare system contributes to the current epidemic of obesity. Even though obesity is now considered a disease, many doctors still consider it an eating problem and ignore the possibility that there are underlying metabolic issues. I have seen countless patients who had gone from doctor to doctor looking for answers, and were given the same advice by them all: eat less. It is important for the healthcare practitioner to sit down and talk to the obese patient. The practitioner needs to look and listen for clues indicating hormones out of balance—excess adrenaline, insulin, cortisol, or estrogen, or a low-functioning thyroid. What drugs is the person taking? What are the person's eating and drinking habits and activity level?

One of my patients—a classic if somewhat extreme case of creative type ADHD—weighed 420 pounds when he first came to see me. The amount of adrenaline required to cause that amount of weight gain also provoked other problems, such as alcoholism and fibromyalgia. This man's previous doctors had accused him of eating too much, even though he assured them he wasn't. If they had been listening to him, the fact that he was not a big eater would have been the first clue that he had a hormone problem, not an eating problem.

This patient presented as a textbook case of imbalanced hormones in terms of both his history and his appearance. Not only was his body pouring out insulin, cortisol, and adrenaline, his excess fat was producing a lot of estrogen, which is a lipogenic (fat-creating) hormone, causing him to put on fat around his hips, thighs, and buttocks. His high insulin level put on weight around his middle. I was not surprised to find that his thyroid level was low-normal, which contributed to fat deposition everywhere.

After I started treating him with progesterone cream, a meal plan designed to reduce adrenaline, and thyroid supplementation, his adrenaline level dropped, his fibromyalgia disappeared, and he reported feeling better than at any time in his life. After losing 240 pounds, he got down to a waist size of 32 inches. He had been suicidal when I first met him, and at the age of 47 he had never had a single date in his life. After he lost weight and improved his well-being, he started dating, got engaged, and is now happily married.

TELOMERES AND AGING

Could reducing excess adrenaline actually increase one's life span? It appears to be so. Currently a lot of research is examining the relationship between the length of telomeres—nucleotide sequences found on the tips of chromosomes—and aging. The evidence suggests that people with shortened telomeres may have a higher incidence of heart attacks and cancer.

A biotech pharmaceutical company developed a drug that could prevent the shortening of telomeres. To avoid the five to ten years of FDA-required trials costing hundreds of millions of dollars, the company sold the rights for this substance to a nutraceutical company. The supplement, called TA-65, originally sold for $24,000 for a year's worth. This cost has now been reduced to $2,400 to $8,000 per year, depending on dosage.

Studies have shown that TA-65 increases the enzyme telomerase, which protects telomeres from getting shorter. It is most effective on rapidly dividing cells, such as the skin, the immune system, and the GI tract. The concern, of course, is that cancer cells are also rapidly dividing cells, but as yet this has not been noted as a problem.

The results so far are anecdotal. Moreover, the doctors who are selling this substance are "anti-aging" specialists, so most of their clients could be taking bio-identical hormones as well, which may also be influencing the way the clients look and feel.

Allow me to present an alternative, less expensive approach. It has clearly been demonstrated that stress reduces telomere size, while reducing stress increases telomere size. (This may be why people dealing with large amounts of stress have a higher mortality rate.)

Adrenaline is closely associated with stress, and reducing adrenaline is known to lower stress levels. Exercise is one way of burning up adrenaline, and exercise has also been shown to increase telomere length in people who have elevated stress levels. Meditation, another stress reducer, has similarly been found to increase telomere length. However, why not reduce stress just by lowering excess adrenaline?

INSOMNIA

Insomnia refers to trouble falling asleep, trouble staying asleep, or both. People can have difficulty achieving sound sleep for a variety of reasons, including physical discomfort, emotional issues, and financial problems. However, in my view, excess adrenaline may be insomnia's number one cause.

As we have seen, adrenaline works as both a hormone, affecting a number of bodily functions, and as a neurotransmitter in the brain. People with a high level of adrenaline functioning as a hormone are generally the ones who have trouble falling asleep. These are people with typical type ADHD who as adults might have type A personalities. The extra energy produced by excess adrenaline may prevent them from feeling tired.

The approach to helping these people fall asleep is to prevent the buildup of adrenaline during the day. A regular exercise regimen to burn off excess adrenaline may also be helpful. Those who awaken during the night are often people with creative type ADHD. These are often the people who complain that their mind does not shut off at night. From a survival standpoint, the body always wants to ensure that the brain has enough fuel to function properly. And the creative brain is more active than a normal brain and therefore requires more fuel. If, during the night, the body detects that the brain has used up its fuel, it will release adrenaline to raise the sugar level and the person will wake up. This release of adrenaline most often occurs between 2:30 and 3:00 a.m. and can continue throughout the rest of the night, so the person may keep waking up intermittently or even not be able to fall back to sleep.

If, during the night, the body detects that the brain has used up its fuel, it will release adrenaline to raise the sugar level and the person will wake up.

The release of adrenaline around 2:30 a.m. may cause hot flashes in perimenopausal or menopausal women with creative type ADHD, and may cause both men and women to experience the urge to urinate starting around this time.

The treatment to prevent adrenaline levels from rising during the night is to eat a light low-glycemic snack shortly before bedtime, preceded by the application of progesterone cream.

RESTLESS LEG SYNDROME

Excess adrenaline during the night can also cause restless leg syndrome (RLS), an uncomfortable sensation in the lower extremities coupled with an uncontrollable urge to move them. Some people actually get out of bed and walk around to get relief. The same problem can be observed during the day in people who persistently move one leg up and down while they are sitting or feel the need to pace.

Some people get cramps in their calves or their feet during the night. This is due to adrenaline constricting arteries and cutting off circulation to the muscles. Cold hands and cold feet can similarly be caused by adrenaline constricting blood vessels and impairing blood flow. This is often mistakenly attributed to an underactive thyroid lowering the body temperature.

People with restless leg syndrome very often have associated symptoms also resulting from elevated adrenaline, such as teeth grinding, the need to urinate, and tossing and turning (restless body syndrome), and they often awaken in the morning with low back pain.

Again, treatment involves preventing adrenaline from spiking during the night by applying progesterone cream and then eating a light low-glycemic snack before bed, and possibly exercising during the day to burn up excess adrenaline. Direct application of progesterone cream to the area of the feet or calves that is cramping often brings relief in less than a minute.

HEADACHES

People with excess adrenaline often suffer from frequent headaches. Adrenaline can give rise to muscle tension in different areas of the body. When the tension is localized to the neck—not an uncommon place to feel tension—it can cause traction headaches, also known as tension headaches.

One type of traction headache, called occipital neuritis, is often mistaken for a migraine headache because the pain can be severe. However, a migraine is characterized by a pulsating type of pain, while the pain of occipital neuritis is piercing. It arises at the base of the skull on one side or the other and shoots into the back of the eye on the affected side. The diagnosis can be confirmed by pressing the thumb into the suspected area at the base of the skull, which should be very painful. Applying moist heat to this area usually provides relief; however, preventing muscle tension around the nerve sheath by lowering the adrenaline level is the cure.

I have recommended to patients with tinnitus that they apply progesterone to the back of the neck, and most of them have obtained significant relief.

Muscle tension in the neck can also give rise to tinnitus, which is a ringing in one or both ears. The two vertebral arteries, which run up the back of the neck into the brain, give rise in the neck to the smaller vestibular arteries, one going to each inner ear. It is my theory that tension in the neck muscles can constrict these small blood vessels, causing impairment of circulation to the inner ear and thus causing tinnitus. I have recommended to patients who have tinnitus that they apply progesterone to the back of the neck, and most of them have obtained significant relief.

Another example of localized muscle tension is temporomandibular joint dysfunction (TMJ), a condition that may arise when people grind their teeth or clench their jaw, especially at night. TMJ can be treated with a dental prosthesis or a retainer, or more simply by lowering adrenaline.

Notably, a low progesterone level can cause a headache in three ways. First, a low progesterone level is associated with increased insulin, which can cause hypoglycemia. Hypoglycemia can lead to a hunger headache, often between 3 and 4 p.m. Second, the hypoglycemia can prompt the release of adrenaline, which can cause traction headaches. Third, women with low progesterone levels can get estrogen-induced migraine headaches when they have their periods.

All of the kinds of headaches mentioned in this section respond quickly, sometimes immediately, to transdermal progesterone cream. The following story illustrates the power of this simple treatment:

I was asked to consult on a case of a 15-year-old boy who had been suffering from a persistent, nonstop headache, along with associated muscle tension in his neck, for 18 months. He was exceptionally intelligent and had classic symptoms of mixed type ADHD. Putting these factors together, I was confident that his headache was caused by excess adrenaline. I placed a small amount of over-the-counter progesterone cream on his forearm and on the back of his neck. In about five minutes his headache was 90 percent gone; after 10 minutes, it was 100 percent gone.

ADDICTIONS

As we have seen, a high level of adrenaline creates anxiety, depression, or anger. In order to "chill out," people with excess adrenaline often turn to alcohol, drugs, cigarettes, or some combination of them. Abusive use of these substances can lead to addictions. Regular exercise to burn off excess adrenaline—engaging in sports, going to the gym, jogging, doing hard work outdoors—can help. However, when these people stop the intense physical activity, the tendency to turn again to addictive substances may reappear.

Michael Phelps, the great Olympic swimmer, was on Ritalin for ADHD in his younger years and got into swimming to eliminate the need for it. He burned up so much adrenaline with his swimming that he was able to stop taking the medicine. However, when he cut back on his swimming after the 2008 Beijing Olympics, his adrenaline again built up, and he was caught smoking marijuana—a disappointment to many of his fans and commercial sponsors. However, when one appreciates the power of adrenaline, it's easy to understand that he may have needed something to relax.

It makes sense that people who rely on adrenaline to do their work—professional athletes, executives, law officers, and construction workers, as well as highly creative people such as artists and performers—would turn to drugs or alcohol in their downtime, again, just to relax. Similarly, I suspect that nearly everyone in Alcoholics Anonymous has had problems with too much adrenaline. It is the same with people who smoke two or three packs of cigarettes per day: they need to counteract the adrenaline in their systems.

From a health standpoint, of course, smokers are setting themselves up for a multitude of serious conditions, including COPD, lung cancer, and heart disease. The huge number of people who are on prescription psychoactive drugs or who drink too much or use marijuana to relax all pose a significant danger to others and to themselves if they drive while under the influence. The cost of excess adrenaline to the healthcare system and to society at large is incalculable. And what about people in our prisons? An estimated 85 percent of people in prison have had problems related to drugs and alcohol. Could excess adrenaline be contributing to the fact that so many former prisoners wind up back in prison?

The cost of excess adrenaline to the healthcare system and to society at large is incalculable.

When it comes to standard methods for dealing with addiction, the success rate of detox or rehab programs is not impressive. Yet detox centers are thriving. Some of the most expensive detox facilities are located in Southern California, where I live. I have approached a number of these centers, including the Betty Ford Center in my hometown, Rancho Mirage, but found that none of them expressed interest in utilizing an approach that addressed the underlying cause of their clients' addictions.

The Church of Scientology—whether or not one agrees with their philosophy—deserves credit for advocating that people get off psychoactive drugs. However, they rely on outside "wellness" doctors to do this. I pointed out to some Scientology executives that doctors will not take patients off a psychoactive drug unless they are given a reasonable alternative to help deal with the patient's illness. I proposed that they set up their own clinics and staff them with doctors trained to lower adrenaline levels, and I offered to provide consulting services. They, too, were not interested.

The problem, of course, is that most doctors, including wellness doctors, do not appreciate the causative role of adrenaline in addiction. Reducing the adrenaline levels of people with substance addictions actually takes away their need to drink or do drugs. Using bio-identical progesterone correctly, people can often gradually give up psychoactive drugs with few or no withdrawal symptoms. But at present there is not enough incentive for healthcare administrators to change the status quo. The medical system is a multi-trillion-dollar-a-year industry that thrives on disease and illness. Nothing in healthcare is going to change until people get angry enough to demand it.

Reducing the adrenaline levels of people with substance addictions actually takes away their need to drink or do drugs.

URINARY URGENCY AND BED-WETTING

Urinary urgency, or "overactive bladder," that experience of "when you have to go, you have to go," is yet another condition caused by adrenaline. Adrenaline increases perfusion through the kidneys, which in turn increases urinary output. At the same time, adrenaline gives people the urge to urinate.

People who are releasing excess adrenaline all day and all night often experience this kind of urinary urgency. They frequently experience dribbling on the way to the bathroom—a condition called urgency incontinence. An article in the September 16, 2010 issue of the *New England Journal of Medicine* that reviewed the many pharmaceutical and surgical approaches to incontinence, not surprisingly, said nothing about adrenaline as a causative factor.

Urgency incontinence is not to be confused with stress incontinence, a condition found mostly in women whereby they lose muscle control around the urethra. Under stress, such as coughing, sneezing, or laughing, urine leaks out. Even though incontinence is not a bladder problem, women with this condition are often given drugs to relax the bladder, such as Detrol or Ditropan, which are ineffective and have anticholinergic side effects (such as dry mouth, constipation, and glaucoma). Or they receive surgical treatment, such as placement of a vaginal mesh, which has been known to cause severe complications. The latest approach is to inject Botox into the bladder muscles. However, incontinence is not caused by a Botox deficiency. Moreover, Botox is so effective at preventing incontinence that women can wind up with the opposite problem and require catheter placement for three months until the drug wears off.

However, stress incontinence can be completely eliminated, usually in three to six days, using intravaginal bio-identical testosterone cream in conjunction with doing Kegel exercises. I discuss this in more detail in my books *The Miracle of Bio-Identical Hormones* and *The Platt Protocol for Hormone Balancing.*

The release of adrenaline at night to raise the sugar level to fuel the brain is very often the cause of nighttime urination.

Many people have problems with nocturia (nighttime urination); some have to get up three or four times a night. This condition is often blamed on drinking too many fluids, prostate problems, heart problems, or having a "small bladder." However, the release of adrenaline at night to raise the sugar level to fuel the brain is very often the cause.

A child who has problems with enuresis (bed-wetting) almost always has ADHD. In fact, a pediatric urologist shared with me that the correlation between bed-wetting and ADHD is widely acknowledged in his field. I have observed that bed-wetting seems to occur almost exclusively in children who have a creative type (right-brained) component to their ADHD. This is not surprising, since the right brain is more active, even at night, so more adrenaline is released during the night, creating the urge to urinate.

Bed-wetting seems to occur almost exclusively in children who have a creative type (right-brained) component to their ADHD.

The pediatric urologist also told me that the primary treatment for bed-wetting in children was Vasopressin, a powerful antidiuretic hormone. I expressed surprise at the time that the FDA would allow this. To their credit, the FDA did wake up to the dangers of using this drug in children and has since disallowed it. However, this raises the question: what drugs might these doctors be prescribing now?

Again, to my way of thinking, the urinary issues just discussed are all about adrenaline. Children with excess adrenaline can have a problem with bed-wetting, and adults with excess adrenaline will get up at night to urinate. Lowering the adrenaline level in both children and adults can bring dramatic improvement in this condition.

HOW ADRENALINE DOMINANCE PRESENTS: PATIENT OBSERVATIONS

Excess adrenaline rarely causes a single condition. It is more likely to manifest as several conditions. The particular array of conditions tends to be unique to each patient, and in general, the number and severity of the conditions may increase as the years go by. Thus the following key points can be made:

1. The effects of excess adrenaline frequently start in childhood and progress throughout adulthood.

2. A person often has a combination of the "good," "bad," and "ugly" effects of adrenaline.

3. Everyone is different in terms of how they react to excess adrenaline.

4. Everyone is the same in terms of the dramatic relief they experience from reducing adrenaline.

These points are illustrated in two letters from patients that follow.

I have found that excess adrenaline is almost always associated with a low progesterone level. Low progesterone would account for the history of severe menstrual cramps described in the first letter. I suspect that this woman's severe constipation was a manifestation of irritable bowel syndrome exacerbated by low thyroid function. The almost miraculous change in her demeanor and feelings she describes can only be attributed to a decrease in her adrenaline.

Patient K.B.

November 3, 2009

Good morning everyone,

This past week has been like moving from living in black and white to waking up each day [to living] in color …. The shades of grey are slipping away more and more each day and are being replaced equally by a brilliance of colors. That is the best description I can share.

Today is the last day that I will be taking both Lamictal and Seroquel. Good riddance! I woke up today realizing something BIG is happening and I'd best keep a record of it!

I am now convinced that the better cause of my turbulent childhood was my imbalance of hormones. What I can remember of my childhood (and that is not much) that directly contributes to my areas of concern today are, but are not limited to, the following:

Constant constipation with periods between bowel movements of 7–10 days and sometimes longer, throughout my entire life. Horrible menstrual cramps with clotting. Inability to concentrate; an inability to relax and "be myself" at any time, even when alone. Nervous, self-doubt, and on and on….

I thought that I would share my journal entry for today, which prompted this e-mail:

Today is Monday Nov. 3, 2009. I woke up today, after an extremely restful night, in no pain, energized, alert, clear headed, light spirited, calm, no pressure in my head, clear eyes, excited (and I am sure there are more adjectives that apply here) for the very first time that I can recall in my entire life. I know that Dr. Platt said that this would happen, but I walked out scared shitless that

"I" would be right and that "Dr. Platt" would be wrong in my case. (After all, I sat through that meeting in my numbed, lethargic, toxic state, hearing the words as they "bounced" off of my head.) I was sure that it would not happen to me. I didn't even know what good "feelings" to expect or how to recognize them if they "popped up"! I actually asked myself, "How will I know that I am feeling better?" I didn't know how horrible I felt. I just didn't know . . . and the journaling goes on.

These are my good reasons to journal. I always want to reference how bad I felt so I would never forget again. Our minds are designed to eliminate bad pain, but this bad pain always needs to be remembered at a safe distance and in a safe place, in the way of a reference point.

I initially came to you for severe constipation and incontinence as well as rapid hair loss, just as my mother had. My remarkable improvement in one short week, in all of these areas and more, additionally gives me hope that my hair will hang in there (no pun intended) for a few more years than my mother's did.
With great appreciation,
K.B.

The patient who wrote the following letter consulted with doctors in five specialties at the Mayo Clinic, who put her through an extensive workup. Even though they eliminated lupus as one of her diagnoses, not one of them suggested that she taper off any of her nine medications, even the ones prescribed for lupus.

In general, doctors hesitate to eliminate a drug that another doctor has prescribed. This is one reason why traditional medicine so often fails at getting patients well.

Patient C.R.
November 16, 2009
Dear Dr. Platt,

I am writing to express my deep gratitude and appreciation for all that you have done for me in assisting me to basically turn my life around. When I first came to you as a new patient for treatment approximately 3 months ago, I had just been to the Mayo Clinic in Scottsdale, AZ, for an extensive series of evaluations by five doctors, who ordered a comprehensive workup of diagnostic tests for fibromyalgia, systemic lupus, and multiple health issues: interstitial cystitis; irritable bowel syndrome; fibromyalgia; peripheral neuropathy; sleep disorder; anxiety; depression; and chronic fatigue. I was a mess!

Fortunately, I found out at Mayo that I did not have lupus, which had been misdiagnosed by my rheumatologist in Hawaii, who had prescribed Lyrica, Prednisone, and hydroxychloroquine for my pain and inflammation and to suppress my immune system. When I came to you last August, I was not only taking these medications, but also Lexapro, Wellbutrin, Ambien, Sonata, Detrol, and Vicodin—all prescribed by different MDs in Hawaii as well. I was so exhausted all of the time. I could barely get out of bed! I felt like my health was spiraling downwards and that I had no recourse but to seek an alternative approach from one of the most highly respected medical professionals in your field. That is why I sought you out. And, not surprisingly, during that first consultation with you I realized that all of the medications with their respective side effects were actually poisoning me and making me worse.

When you asked me to wean myself off the medications

and begin taking bio-identical hormones and change my meal plan, along with an entire program of natural nutritional supplements tailored for my specific needs, I was ready—not only because I was desperate to feel better and felt literally like I was dying—but because you really took the time during that first consultation to explain to me the biochemical mechanisms within my body which were causing, for example, the fibromyalgia and related disorders. You helped me to understand my body from a holistic approach, and therefore be open to treatment that was natural instead of chemical and would actually help my body heal itself. Your nutritional counseling, as well, helped me immensely to develop healthier eating habits that have supported my healing process and continue to make a huge difference in my overall well-being.

So, as you can imagine, I am happy to say that your approach has worked! Since I have been off the medications for the last approximately 3 months and using the bio-identical hormones and changing the way I eat along with the supplements, my whole life is different. In fact, I really feel that your first consultation and subsequent discussions we have had, as well as your medical literature, have been a real wake-up call for me, and have actually saved my life! Before I came in to see you for the first time, I truly was feeling progressively worse and worse all of the time while on all of those medications, like I had constant flu-like symptoms. I was losing hope for any chance at living a normal, healthy life again. I would look at myself, a former model, and it appeared as though I was aging almost before my eyes…. But now, after only 3 months, not only have my life and health turned around, but I also feel and look more vibrant and alive than I have in years! My energy is back better than ever, and everyone from family to friends I have not seen in years keep asking me "What happened?" "What have you done to yourself?" They keep telling me I "look younger," which of course I love!

I am so happy that I took that first step to come in to see you and allow you to convince me to "think out of the box" (my term, not yours, but I feel it is appropriate)! Coming from a family of doctors and medical professionals, that was a big step to take, but again I want to thank you for taking the time and having the compassion and commitment to do what you do for your patients every day. I only wish more doctors would take your approach of not just treating the symptoms, but rather treating and healing the true underlying illness. As your patient, I am a living testimony to the fact that your approach not only works, but also is profoundly successful! Every condition I mentioned is now gone—including the depression, fibromyalgia, interstitial cystitis, stress incontinence, sleep problems, anxiety, irritable bowel syndrome, etc. I am so convinced of this that I have already referred and will continue to refer many beloved friends and family members, and even clients, to you from all over the world that are desperately in need of an alternative and more natural, holistic approach to the traditional medical model of using drugs to treat the symptoms (which is not working for them, either!). It is an honor and privilege to do so, because I feel that you have helped me to get my life back, and for that I am eternally grateful!

CHAPTER 7 | EXCESS ADRENALINE: THE UGLY

What I refer to as the "ugly" conditions caused by excess adrenaline represent hyperadrenalism's more devastating effects. These are the illnesses that I feel have the most significant impact on a person's quality of life. Like the conditions already discussed, all these maladies are generally considered incurable. Yet every one of them can be "cured" by addressing its root cause, which in every case has to do with too much adrenaline.

There is an art to helping a patient get well. It starts with having a basic knowledge of hormones, since they control every system in the body. It also involves sitting down with the patient and listening to what he or she is saying. Ninety percent of a diagnosis should be based on this conversation.

There is an art to helping a patient get well. It starts with a basic knowledge of hormones and also involves sitting down with the patient and listening to what he or she is saying.

FIBROMYALGIA

Fibromyalgia has had a singularly unimpressive history from a clinical standpoint. For a long time, half the doctors in

America did not believe this condition existed; the other half believed it was a real condition, yet it sometimes took 20 years to diagnose, and even then doctors could only say, "There's nothing we can do for it." Although conventional medicine considers it incurable, fibromyalgia can often be eliminated in anywhere from three days to three weeks by reducing the patient's level of adrenaline. Most people with this condition have other adrenaline-induced problems as well. These, too, can be eliminated along with the fibromyalgia.

Even though millions of people suffer in various degrees from this condition, and tremendous research has been done on its etiology, modern medicine still cannot pinpoint its causation, although several theories have been proposed. For example, the latest research theorizes that fibromyalgia has a neurogenic origin having to do with the amplification of pain signals. Researchers have noticed disturbances in the levels of neurotransmitters that either facilitate pain awareness or prevent it—which, of course, suggests that drugs that affect these neurotransmitters can help. (Notably, researchers have made similar findings in a number of chronic pain conditions, such as irritable bowel syndrome, TMJ, and interstitial cystitis—all of which are discussed in this book.) A television advertisement for the drug Lyrica, for example, states that fibromyalgia is caused by stimulation of overactive nerve tissue. These are classic examples of how drug companies control how medicine is practiced.

One of the problems with evidence-based medicine is that one never knows what's real. Pharmaceutical companies sponsor many of the studies, and it is well known that their financial support often influences the researchers and their results. This is why I feel more comfortable with observation-based medicine. To me it seems logical that if a medical practitioner treating patients with a particular approach can successfully predict the outcome in almost 100 percent of cases, this should fulfill the criteria for evidence-based medicine. In this regard, the fact that I have eliminated fibromyalgia in the vast majority of my patients who were suffering from it should give credibility to my approach.

If a medical practitioner treating patients with a particular approach can successfully predict the outcome in almost 100 percent of cases, this should fulfill the criteria for evidence-based medicine.

Fibromyalgia is indicated by two major symptoms: pain and fatigue. The pain of fibromyalgia, I believe, is due to a buildup of lactic acid in muscles and tendon sheaths. This pain is similar to "muscle burn" experienced by athletes from working out. Muscle burn is caused by the buildup of lactic acid. The difference between muscle burn and fibromyalgia is that after athletes work out, their muscles usually relax, possibly because they have burned up a lot of adrenaline. As those muscles relax, circulation moving through them clears out the excess lactic acid, thereby eliminating the pain. But people who have fibromyalgia often find it hard to relax. Their muscles remain tense, which compresses the venules of the blood circulation system and the small vessels of the lymphatic circulation system, both of which normally carry lactic acid out of the muscles. As a result, the acid stays in the muscles and in tendon sheaths, and the pain persists.

This constant tensing of muscles, even through the night,

causes fatigue, and at times, severe fatigue. Patients often awaken with low back pain, upper back pain, or pain on the side of one hip. At night they may also tense their jaw, causing TMJ (temporomandibular joint dysfunction), or grind their teeth. The persistent tensing of muscles uses up nutrients that support muscle function (ATP, CoQ10, carnitine, magnesium, etc.), so the recovery from using certain muscle groups may be very slow.

The diagnosis of fibromyalgia is not difficult, even though it so often goes unrecognized. Eighteen pressure points on the body have been identified, the compression of which elicits pain in patients with fibromyalgia. It is not unusual for medical practitioners to conclude that what they are seeing is an autoimmune condition (which it is not) or to refer the patient to a rheumatologist because they think it is an inflammatory condition (which it is not). Because of the associated fatigue, people with fibromyalgia are also frequently diagnosed as having chronic fatigue syndrome. However, chronic fatigue syndrome is most likely viral in origin and is associated with low-grade fevers and swollen lymph glands. Of course, some people may have both conditions.

There are no laboratory tests to directly diagnose fibromyalgia, but several tests help rule out other conditions. For example, the results of the C-reactive protein and sedimentation rate tests are elevated in inflammatory conditions but should be normal in fibromyalgia. The ANA (antinuclear antibiodies) test, which screens for autoimmune conditions like lupus, should also be normal in fibromyalgia.

There is one lab test, however, that offers indirect evidence for fibromyalgia. This is the morning plasma cortisol test, which can indicate an elevated adrenaline level. The standard "normal" level (up to 19.4) for this test I believe is misleading; instead, I feel that any level greater than 11.5 suggests an overproduction of adrenaline. This is because the normal ranges for many lab tests were originally established by testing the blood of medical students. Because adrenaline enhances intelligence and medical students tend to be intelligent, their a.m. cortisol levels would have likely been relatively high.

In my view, there are two main causes of fibromyalgia. The less common of the two is related to the displacement of the first cervical vertebra (C1), also called the atlas. The atlas sits at the top of the cervical spine, directly supporting the skull, and nerves pass through a hole in the atlas on the way to the brain. It is not uncommon for the atlas to be displaced when there has been a neck injury caused by, for instance, a whiplash or falling off a horse or bicycle. Displacement of the atlas can lead to irritation of the nerves passing through it, which can cause headaches, neck pain, upper shoulder pain, or arm pain. The pain can cause muscles to tense up, resulting in a buildup of lactic acid, which exacerbates the pain further.

The importance of considering this cause of fibromyalgia is that it is best treated by chiropractors specially trained to manipulate the atlas either manually or by using an activator. (See the website www.nucca.org for names of chiropractors in various locations trained in this method.) Alternatively, specially trained orthodontists can supply a prosthesis that may realign the atlas.

However, the more common cause of fibromyalgia, in my view, is the internalization of anger, associated with excess adrenaline. Adrenaline, known as the fight-or-flight hormone, should also be called the rage hormone, or anger hormone. Anger created by this powerful hormone is an intense feeling that, when suppressed, can cause persistent muscle tension with associated pain and fatigue. Because the anger is internalized, many people with fibromyalgia may not even realize that they have anger issues. Interestingly, they occasionally exhibit anger when someone suggests that they have anger issues.

The more common cause of fibromyalgia is internalization of anger associated with excess adrenaline.

The underlying anger can cause persistent tensing of muscles, which constricts circulation and prevents the buildup of lactic acid from being cleared. Eliminating the cause of the anger will, in most cases, eliminate the fibromyalgia, as the following stories of two of my fibromyalgia patients demonstrate. Their stories bring to mind one of my favorite quotes from Wayne Dyer: "Every moment of your life you spend upset, in despair, in anguish, angry, or hurt because of the behavior of anybody else in your life is the moment you have given up control of your life."

A 52-year-old woman with severe fibromyalgia came to see me. When I asked her about anger issues, she said her only known source of anger was her five-month-old puppy, which she had brought to my office with her. She happened to be a perfectionist, and the dog, she said, kept urinating on her carpet. She would not allow the dog to sleep on her bed because she worried he would urinate there. She could not visit her daughter because her daughter had two large dogs. In other words, the puppy was controlling her life. I suggested that since she did not have the temperament to live with a dog, she should give her dog away. Hearing that, she handed the puppy to one of my nurses. When she came back two days later to give some of the dog paraphernalia to the nurse, she commented: "I cannot believe how much better I feel."

A 38-year-old woman came in with severe fibromyalgia. I had seen her six years prior and had diagnosed her then as having fibromyalgia. At that time, our discussion uncovered the fact that the source of her anger was her husband, who was abusive. Since I approach illness by addressing its cause, I recommended that she consider dissolving their relationship. Now she was back, six years later, still with severe fibromyalgia and still with the same husband—who was still abusing her. So again, I suggested that she consider dissolving their relationship because he clearly was not going to change his behavior. One week later she returned—laughing and smiling. Her fibromyalgia was completely gone. She had left her husband.

These two cases represent a type of fibromyalgia that could be called "reactive fibromyalgia," comparable to the condition "reactive depression." However, I suspect that most clinically relevant fibromyalgia is from internalized anger due to excess adrenaline. People with this type of fibromyalgia may have other excess adrenaline problems as well, such as depression, irritable bowel syndrome, or insomnia. They may wind up on multiple medications, which can add to their malaise by causing weight gain, impotence, confusion, additional fatigue, and other symptoms.

For example, a pastor who came to see me was on 15 different medications for treatment of severe fibromyalgia, depression, and sleeping problems. His congregation thought he had Alzheimer's disease because his speech was slurred and he appeared demented—though these were actually side effects from the drugs. I helped him to quickly wean himself off all his medications and also treated the underlying excess adrenaline. His fibromyalgia, depression, slurred voice, cognitive impairment, and insomnia disappeared. His congregation thought a miracle had happened. The next time he came into the office I chided him, "Do you realize that Jesus is getting all the credit for what I did for you?" He looked at me and replied, "Jesus sent me to you." Spoken like a true pastor.

I have seen a number of pastors in my practice. One thing they all had in common is the symptoms of creative type ADHD, which is associated with intelligence and enhanced creativity.

The patient who wrote the following letter found that her fibromyalgia was gone three days after she first came to my office. When I asked how she got better so quickly, she responded that as soon as she had insight as to the cause, she was able to take the steps to eliminate it.

Patient C.C.

My first visit to Dr. Platt was in June of 2003, seven years ago. I suffered from fibromyalgia and chronic fatigue syndrome. I had seen multiple physicians, but none of them ever had a solution for me. It took my last doctor five years to figure out the above problems, and all he did was put me on drugs to mask the problems. I was missing five or six weeks of work at a time.

I went to see Dr. Platt, who took the time to talk and explain that I was not crazy. I did everything he asked. In just days I had more energy, no brain fog, and NO PAIN.

I have not missed one day of work in the last seven years and I have never felt better. Dr. Platt gave me back my life, and I will forever be grateful.

The following letter shows how important it is for patients to understand why they are not well. It is actually part of the healing process.

Patient L.C.

My recent visit with you is still in the forefront of my mind. I have been to many medical doctors, osteopaths, and chiropractors in my 64 years, and I wanted to tell you that the best doctor I have ever had an appointment with is definitely you.

As you know, I was suffering very badly with fibromyalgia. My energy level was nil. The program that you put me on has worked miracles. I no longer have the fibromyalgia pain all over my body. I am no longer falling asleep for two hours after I eat my breakfast and my lunch. I am actually sleeping for seven hours plus each night without waking up five times during the night for a bathroom visit. My energy level has soared!

So now I am back to my old self—busy doing things every day, walking and using a re-bounder. Previously, I was basically a couch potato without energy or motivation to do ANYTHING. I would have low energy crashes and I thought I might have diabetes. Knowing that I had a hormone problem, which has been corrected with natural products, and I don't have a disease, I feel like living my life again.

Please do not stop fighting to help people get well because you're one of the few who do really put people on the right track. I cannot express enough how grateful I am for the work that you do. And thank you, Dr. Platt,

for your continual work to give back lives, even against
all the aggression/oppression you have in your daily life.
Sincerely,
L.C., Ph.D.

CHRONIC INTERSTITIAL CYSTITIS

An estimated 750,000 to 1,000,000 women in the United States suffer from a condition called chronic interstitial cystitis. It often manifests as severe pain in the bladder 24 hours a day, along with uncomfortable burning during urination. Like so many other conditions discussed in this book, it has no known cause and, as a consequence, no known cure. It is most commonly treated with the drug Elmiron, which offers little or no help to the majority of women who use it.

I consider chronic interstitial cystitis another manifestation of adrenaline dominance. As we saw in the section on urinary urgency (in the previous chapter), excess adrenaline can cause not only the urge to urinate but also the need to urinate frequently. However, some women, for one reason or another—perhaps they work as teachers or cashiers—do not have the luxury of being able to run to the bathroom every 20 minutes or so. As a result, they tense up the muscles of the bladder in an attempt to prevent leakage. Any prolonged tensing of muscles can cause lactic acid to build up. This, in turn, can cause both pain in the walls of the bladder and burning upon urination.

Because of the role of lactic acid buildup in chronic interstitial cystitis, I refer to it as fibromyalgia of the bladder. Not surprisingly, it is often associated with fibromyalgia elsewhere in the body.

Because of the role of lactic acid buildup in chronic interstitial cystitis, I refer to it as fibromyalgia of the bladder.

Elimination of this condition makes for an extremely grateful patient. One of my patients had been to doctors all over the world looking for relief. Two weeks after visiting my office, she sent a card thanking me and called me her "miracle doctor." The treatment, needless to say, was simply to lower her adrenaline level.

Trying to educate people who are in a position to change how this condition is treated has been frustrating. As an example, I approached the Interstitial Cystitis Association and offered to write an article for their newsletter about how I treat this condition, but they were not interested. Perhaps they could not fathom that this devastating condition might have a relatively simple solution.

ROAD RAGE

I have included road rage in the "ugly" category because it is a potentially lethal condition, especially if two people with road rage come into contact with one another. People with road rage often tailgate other cars, they tend to drive too fast and make unsafe lane changes, and they certainly antagonize other drivers—especially those who also have road rage. It takes very little imagination to see that these people have an excessive amount of adrenaline. They frequently wind up in anger management classes, although these classes provide little benefit because they do not link the problem with its real cause.

Road rage can have serious consequences. For example, a medical doctor in Los Angeles with excess adrenaline got into a road rage incident with two bicyclists who also had excess adrenaline. The doctor wound up in prison for five years, and both bicycle riders were hospitalized. One of them will never ride a bike again.

Those who have a tendency toward road rage should keep in mind that their driving is monitored by law enforcement personnel who usually have excess adrenaline themselves. When an officer pulls a driver over and tells the driver to get out of the car and lie down on the ground, my recommendation is to do what the officer says. One only has to remember what happened to Rodney King in Los Angeles in 1992. After a long chase by highway patrol officers, he was pulled over and wound up attacking two policemen. He failed to heed their request to lie down, which resulted in his being beaten by over-adrenalized officers, an event that wound up precipitating the infamous Los Angeles Riots.

Of course, the treatment for road rage is to lower adrenaline. The following letter illustrates how quickly this can be accomplished. This 30-year-old gentleman from the San Francisco Bay Area came to see me with only one complaint: anger.

Patient A.W.

Since the first time I rubbed the progesterone cream on my arms I could feel the effects. From that moment on, I have felt an inner calmness that had always seemed to be missing. This was something I had been trying to control for years by using different substances. I feel "normal" again, I should say, I like myself again. The biggest thing for me is driving. As you can imagine, where I live in Silicon Valley there is no shortage of traffic and bad drivers.

Before coming to your office I would have times when I would just choose not to go out because of the devastating effect driving had on my attitude. Sometimes I just wanted to run drivers off the road or honk at them, and I just felt unusually frustrated with the whole experience. I should mention there was a point in my life when I loved to drive. Now, something amazing has happened, I can enjoy driving again. The local driving habits of people, or the lack thereof, haven't changed. I have. It just doesn't bother me anymore. I am amazed, too, when this happens. I think to myself, "Wow, that person just cut me off and that's OK. I am OK with that." Whereas I used to think, "Who in the f#*$ is that a%&#!+?" That is a big difference! I just feel so much better.

I want to thank Dr. Platt and his team for their courage to move forward and really try to heal people during a time when people need it most. I know that there will be/is a lot of resistance, there always is with change, but if I can ever be of help I am here! It has been less than a week since I was there and I am seriously a new person! Before coming in to your office I had been working so hard on the physical and mental parts, but something was still missing. I thank you from the bottom of my heart for filling the missing part. I can now truly live my life.

BIPOLAR DISORDER

In my opinion, understanding how excess adrenaline can affect the body sheds light on the condition known as bipolar disorder. The older term, "manic-depressive disorder," was perhaps a more apt name.

People with this condition go from periods of extreme restlessness and hyperactivity to periods of extreme depression. In the hypomanic phase (a true manic phase is rarely seen outside of an institution), the mind can go extremely fast and the person may exhibit rapid speech or have grandiose ideas. These characteristics are symptoms of excess adrenaline in the brain. This same output of adrenaline, the anger hormone, can lead to depression when the anger is internalized. Subsequently, the adrenaline causes a swing back to euphoria.

There is no way of accurately determining the behaviors through which a bipolar tendency will be expressed. It may be that right-brained patients exhibit more rapid speech and flow of ideas, while left-brained patients may manifest extreme activity. I suspect that both can become severely depressed and suicidal.

I also suspect that everyone with this condition started out with ADHD. People with ADHD can actually be pushed into a bipolar state simply with the use of commonly prescribed antidepressants that are in the norepinephrine reuptake inhibitor (NRI) category, or with stimulants. A partial list of these drugs includes: Wellbutrin, Effexor, Cymbalta, Lyrica, Pristiq, Adderall, Strattera, and Ritalin. The last three are prescribed for ADHD specifically, while the others are commonly used for depression. Bipolar patients are often placed on antidepressants, with Cymbalta and Lyrica added for pain control.

Doctors are giving bipolar patients medications that increase the adrenaline level in the brain when they have too much adrenaline in the brain to begin with.

All of these drugs can increase the amount of adrenaline in the brain. Reminiscent of how doctors often treat type II diabetics with insulin or drugs that increase insulin, the very hormone that causes type II diabetes, doctors are giving bipolar patients medications that increase the adrenaline level in the brain, when they have too much adrenaline in the brain to begin with. Is it any wonder that suicide and sudden death are listed among the side effects of these drugs? As one patient wrote in a brief note:

Patient C.K.
You have taken me off my bipolar drugs and have changed my life. My whole family acknowledges the following: I am more alert. I am walking better with "more life" in my step. My anxiety level is way down and I am no longer sluggish in thought.

How ADHD can convert into a bipolar disorder is illustrated by the case of a 32-year-old patient of mine. He had a history of hyperactivity caused by high adrenaline. In his youth he was active in sports and had trouble focusing in school; as an adult he became a workaholic. His excess adrenaline took away his appetite, which forced the release of even more adrenaline to provide fuel for the body. This also created stress, which led to cortisol production. The cortisol raised his sugar level, leading to the release of insulin, which resulted in hypoglycemia—prompting the output of still more adrenaline. His very high adrenaline caused hypomanic behavior along with episodes of severe depression due to internalization of anger.

When I first met with this patient, he was on four medications: lithium, Depakote, Paxil, and Effexor. The drugs caused him to gain 65 pounds, which added to his depression, along with brain fog. I put him on a program to lower his adrenaline and wean him off all his psychoactive medications. His bipolar behavior disappeared along with his weight gain. He underwent a remarkable transformation, attesting to the ability of the body to heal itself when the underlying cause of the problem is addressed.

Part of the protocol I recommend for treating bipolar disorder is natural bio-identical progesterone cream. Because progesterone is a natural antidepressant that affects most, if not all, of the neurotransmitters in the brain, using it helps patients to wean themselves off their antidepressant drugs.

One woman who came to see me had been diagnosed with bipolar disorder and was on Lyrica, Cymbalta, Effexor, and Wellbutrin. All four drugs are NRIs. NRI drugs increase the level of norepinephrine—a hormone that acts similarly to adrenaline—in the brain. For someone whose adrenaline level in the brain is already raised, taking NRIs can have tragic consequences.

The woman was also in her first trimester of pregnancy. I advised her that if she wanted to maintain the pregnancy, she should go "cold turkey" off her medications to avoid damage to the fetus. She abruptly stopped all medications while applying progesterone cream every one to two hours and did not have a single withdrawal symptom. Needless to say, her bipolar disorder also disappeared.

A Canadian patient who drove all the way from Manitoba to Southern California to see me shared that she had been on 43 medications at one time or another for her bipolar problem and had been institutionalized numerous times for this disorder. Obviously, the drugs were not solving her problem. I helped her wean herself off her medications and prescribed for her high doses of progesterone cream. Not only did she return to feeling normal, she was able to go out and get a job for the first time in 10 years.

When she visited the doctor who had been treating her for years, he didn't even recognize her. It was the first time he had seen her wearing makeup. Prior to this visit she would drag herself out of bed and didn't have the energy to apply makeup. She told him how wonderful she felt off of her medications and on hormones. The doctor promptly scolded her and fired her as a patient. This was not surprising, since she threatened this doctor's approach to treating patients.

Another woman, aged 42, had been diagnosed with bipolar disorder, plus type II diabetes and hypertension. At the time I first saw her, she was on the following daily medications—an example of gross mistreatment of a patient, yet, surprisingly, still within the guidelines of the "standard of care":

> Insulin – 90 units (an extremely high level)
> Seroquel – 25 mg
> Abilify – 5 mg
> Lexapro – 30 mg
> Ritalin – 30 mg
> Provigil – 200 mg
> Metformin – 2000 mg
> Neurontin – 600 mg
> Citrical – 2 tablets

Aspirin – 325 mg
Nexium – 40 mg
Atenolol – 50 mg
Ranitidine – 75 mg
Lipitor – 40 mg
Tricor – 145 mg
Xenical – 120 mg
Lotensin – 20 mg
Provera – 10 mg
Niaspan – 2 capsules
Synthroid – 88 mcg

I eliminated every one of her medications except the thyroid (Synthroid). Her brain fog disappeared. Her sugar level normalized, as did her blood pressure. Her cholesterol actually went down when she was off the Lipitor and Niaspan, and she lost 65 pounds.

Certainly, treating patients with psychoactive disorders can be complex and should not be taken lightly. Reducing adrenaline and weaning off psychoactive drugs may not be suitable for every patient. That said, what I do know is that, given the choice, most patients prefer to treat the cause of their problem and not be subjected to a drug or drugs that can have toxic side effects. In the case of patients diagnosed with bipolar disorder, it is certainly worth considering whether the issue is an underlying hormonal dysfunction that could be treated naturally with the right diet and with bio-identical progesterone.

Until fairly recently, the diagnosis of bipolar disorder in children was virtually nonexistent. Today, over 1 million children have been diagnosed with this condition. The main manifestations seem to be hyperactivity, disruptive behavior, extreme mood swings, and anger issues—all suggestive, of course, of excess adrenaline. These children are often placed on powerful psychoactive drugs, many of which the FDA has not approved for use in children.

Today, over 1 million children have been diagnosed with bipolar disorder, even though they fail to demonstrate the classic signs of severe mood swings.

While high levels of adrenaline can explain all of the behaviors these children exhibit, making that observation is not cost efficient for the business of medicine. Many psychiatrists are compensated only if they prescribe a drug. Once a child is started on an antipsychotic, the psychiatrist has a built-in patient for years to come. Primary care doctors are reluctant to prescribe these types of drugs, and certainly will not take the responsibility of discontinuing them.

My personal view is that the school killings of recent years as well as teenage suicides may have involved young people on these drugs whose side effects have caused these tragic episodes. Although gun legislation may be of benefit, it might be even more effective to limit the prescription of these powerful drugs to children.

A poignant example of the problem with false diagnostic labels, as well as the failure of the medical establishment to understand how hormones affect mental health, is the story of a four-year-old girl, Rebecca Riley. On December 13, 2006, Rebecca died of an overdose of drugs given to her for bipolar disorder, prescribed by a doctor who had never examined her. In 2010, her parents, in separate trials, were found guilty of murder, and both received life sentences. Their crime: deliberately overdosing their daughter.

Her doctor had prescribed excessively high doses of three psychoactive drugs—Depakote 750 mg per day, Seroquel 200 mg per day, and clonidine 0.35 mg per day—based not on examining Rebecca but on the mother's reports of Rebecca's behavior. Interestingly, both the doctor and the mother agreed, in interviews before the trials, that Rebecca most likely did not have bipolar disorder, even though she had been diagnosed with it.

The state of Massachusetts neglected to file charges against the doctor. It is hard to fathom why the doctor was held blameless for Rebecca's death, and why the pharmacists were not reprimanded for refilling the prescriptions for Rebecca almost every other day. In my opinion, every person associated with her care shares the blame for her death: her parents, the doctor, the pharmacists, the staff at her school, and social services. Her death, I feel, could have been prevented had the medical profession been aware of the relationship between hormones and ADHD.

It has been noted that bipolar disorder runs in families. This makes sense since children inherit their hormones from their parents. I would guess that the parents of children who are given a bipolar diagnosis both have ADHD. Indeed, most of the patients I have seen with bipolar disorders have the signs and symptoms I recognize as creative type ADHD. In other words, they have a lot of adrenaline in the brain.

The treatment for bipolar disorder that I have found repeatedly effective consists of the patient utilizing the proper dose of progesterone cream, following the correct meal plan, and weaning himself or herself off any bipolar medications he or she is taking.

HYPEREMESIS GRAVIDARUM

It is not unusual for pregnant women to experience morning sickness during the first three months of pregnancy. This nausea and vomiting is caused by estrogen when progesterone, the hormone that normally blocks the effects of estrogen, is inadequate. At the start of the second trimester, the placenta starts putting out large amounts of progesterone, which normally eliminates the nausea and vomiting.

However, some women continue to vomit through their entire pregnancy, a condition known as hyperemesis gravidarum. Not being a gynecologist, I have not seen women in my practice at the time they exhibited this condition. But a number of my women patients report having had this problem during their pregnancies.

These women go into the second trimester with their brains starved for fuel, so their bodies are pouring out adrenaline to raise their sugar levels.

I have noted that the majority of these women have creative type ADHD, which means their brains require more fuel than a "normal" brain. Most of these women are progesterone-deficient to begin with. As a result, they experience fairly intense nausea and vomiting in the first trimester due to unopposed estrogen. They go into the second trimester with their brains starved for fuel, so their bodies are pouring out adrenaline to raise their sugar levels. Unfortunately, this outpouring of adrenaline also induces nausea and vomiting and suppresses the appetite. To exacerbate matters, these women are still putting out large amounts of estrogen, which may also contribute to the nausea and vomiting.

A review article titled "Nausea and Vomiting in Pregnancy" in the October 14, 2010 issue of the *New England Journal of Medicine* says that "the cause of nausea and vomiting in pregnancy is unclear." However, knowing how adrenaline affects the body provides a reasonable explanation of the cause. We know that in certain stressful situations, when the body is likely to produce excess adrenaline, some people experience nausea and vomiting. Examples include performers just before going on stage, professional athletes before going out on the field, and trial attorneys before giving their opening remarks. So overproduction of adrenaline is likely a key factor in women with hyperemesis gravidarum also.

I suspect that giving women suffering from this condition high doses of bio-identical progesterone via vaginal suppositories, along with transdermal progesterone cream, would significantly relieve their symptoms. If nutrition with low-glycemic carbohydrates, either orally (if possible) or via tube feedings, is added, the problem could possibly be eliminated in 24 to 48 hours.

Three other obstetrical complications that also seem related to high adrenaline are preeclampsia, toxemia of pregnancy, and gestational diabetes. Both preeclampsia and toxemia of pregnancy, which are extremely serious, often necessitating early termination of the pregnancy, are associated with hypertension. It seems reasonable that adrenaline and insulin are causing the rise in blood pressure. I also suspect that women with these complications are not producing a sufficient amount of progesterone during their pregnancy. Adrenaline and insulin presumably play key roles in gestational diabetes just like they do in regular diabetes, as discussed in the previous chapter.

At the time of this writing, the FDA has just approved use

of a synthetic progestin to prevent premature births. The cost of this drug is about $1,500 per week. The good news is that compounding pharmacies can provide the identical preparation for about $95 per week. The bad news is that the FDA has made it illegal for compounding pharmacies to compound it. However, there is still a silver lining to this story. Physicians can offer their patients an even better option, namely, bio-identical progesterone in the form of vaginal suppositories and topical cream. The FDA cannot block compounding pharmacies from dispensing bio-identical progesterone suppositories or cream because drug companies do not provide them. Bio-identical progesterone is natural and does not cause the serious side effects that synthetic progestins cause. It is also the least expensive as well as the most effective option.

CYCLICAL VOMITING SYNDROME

Cyclical vomiting syndrome, which is similar to hyperemesis gravidarum, is another condition for which the medical establishment cannot identify a cause. One of my patients, aged 47, had this condition. He told me that every morning of his life he would wake up and vomit. When he was a child, every time he got excited, he would start vomiting and couldn't stop and would have to be hospitalized. To my way of thinking, the only possible explanation for this type of vomiting is adrenaline.

On his first visit he sat across the desk from me, clenching the arms of his chair. It was fairly easy to observe that this man was pouring out adrenaline. I applied some progesterone cream to his forearm, and in less than ten minutes he leaned back in his chair and stated that in his entire life he had never felt so good.

In the six years (as of this writing) since his first visit, he has not had one episode of vomiting. The letter he sent to me clearly delineates the agony he suffered from hyperadrenalism and the effectiveness of treating excess adrenaline with bio-identical progesterone cream.

For all those who have not experienced the symptoms of ADHD, there are absolutely no words to describe how bad, truly bad, life was before....

I first came to Dr. Platt a year and a half ago. I had been on a nine-month merry-go-round of treatments, tests, and scans, all to no avail. Some $18,000 later, an entire staff of doctors could not tell me what was wrong with me.

I was suffering from fibromyalgia. Every single inch of my body hurt. I could not get out of bed in the morning without extreme pain, I mean PAIN.

*When I opened Dr. Platt's book (*The Miracle of Bio-Identical Hormones*), I found all of my life's agonies described on the pages in front of me. What makes me this way and how to fix it, all right there in black and white.*

I had just lost my job due in part to all these symptoms. My new bride of a year and a half was packing her bags, and frankly I was seriously considering jumping off a bridge.

I now know that my adrenal glands are very active, and the one thing that a CT scan showed me is that my adrenal glands are three times larger than the average person's.

After reading Chapter 15 I realized that I have ADHD. How someone can remain undiagnosed at 47 years of age baffles me.

The effect that adrenaline has on so many parts of the body simply amazes me—how it affects hypoglycemia & blood sugar, the endless cycle of adrenaline versus sugar.

In Chapter 15 Dr. Platt addresses adrenaline and its effects on the body in many ways. I counted 27 in just this one chapter.

Adrenaline was killing me....

My wife and I made an appointment to see Dr. Platt. Feeling at the end of our rope, we booked the flights to California.

My mood swings were out of control at this point. Like a clock's pendulum going tick-tock-tick-tock, mine was going: aggression, depression, aggression, depression....

We sat across the desk from Dr. Platt, ranting and raving about all the symptoms, all the tests and aggravations. My wife and I often speak simultaneously, so the doc was getting more than his fill apparently.

"Do you want all this to go away?" he asked me in the most sincere way, like he just fixed people's lives every day. Thirty years of agony and this man says, "DO YOU WANT THIS TO GO AWAY?"

He took progesterone cream and spread it down the length of my forearm. "Now rub that in," he said.

We conversed a while, looked at some blood tests, etc. Ten minutes or so passed. He says, "How do you feel?"

The first thing that came to mind was what I was not feeling....

No adrenaline....

I was calm.

I was sitting still, perfectly still....

ADHD is a hyperactivity disorder. This comes from too much adrenaline. Too much adrenaline attaching to over 15 million neuro-receptors in the brain equals aggression.

Waiting too long in line......Aggression
The waitress forgot my drink......Aggression
Someone didn't live up to my expectations......
Aggression
My life has always been a battle to calm the aggression....
He put that cream on my arm and it was all gone.... Every single symptom GONE.

In the days following I noticed:
No more vomiting in the morning.
No more debilitating fibromyalgia.
No more afternoon fatigue.

Most of all, I am CALM today. It's great to just sit still....

Every single symptom gone in 10 minutes....
What can I tell you about my friend, Dr. Platt?

He has shaken the medical community with his knowledgeable, brutal honesty about how medicine is practiced in our society, how power is abused by our drug manufacturers. He questions the ideas of practitioners who treat the symptoms of disease, not the underlying problem. Make the symptom go away and you're OK.

The understanding this man has of bio-identical hormones and the human body's reaction to hormone imbalance is astounding.

There is no doubt about it! This man saved my life. Not only am I alive today, but I have a quality of life that 30 years of medical treatment and antidepressants could not give me.

I could write a book about all the correct analyses Dr. Platt makes in Chapter 15 about how hormones affect ADHD, HOW ADRENALINE AFFECTS OUR BODIES. I AM LIVING PROOF THAT EVERYTHING THIS MAN SAYS IS TRUE!

No, It's Not a Miracle
It's Dr. Platt

AUTISM

I have not had much personal experience with patients who have autism. But based on what I know about the condition, I strongly suspect that excess adrenaline is involved. Since the incidence of autism is rising, it is becoming increasingly important to recognize this disorder and understand healthy approaches to treating it.

I feel that autism may be an extreme form of creative type ADHD. Autistic children can be extremely intelligent—some of them have been known to memorize a phonebook. At the same time, exceedingly high levels of adrenaline in the brain could be the reason they find it difficult to communicate. They might be shrinking away from sensory input, including eye contact, in order to decrease the amount of stimulus to their over-adrenalized brains.

Autism may be an extreme form of creative type ADHD.

My approach to treating these children would be to use the protocol described in this book: transdermal progesterone cream to help control insulin and adrenaline, and a diet that includes large amounts of low-glycemic carbohydrates, especially green vegetables, in order to provide a steady supply of fuel for the brain. Once adrenaline is lowered, the mind can stop racing. Without the over-stimulation from sensory input, the children might be able to communicate more effectively. In addition, I would recommend certain supplements, including digestive enzymes to help with digesting the vegetables, coconut oil to provide additional fuel for the brain, vitamin D3, and a B vitamin supplement.

Several of my patients who were mothers of autistic children followed this protocol for their children and saw dramatic improvement. One of these mothers included the following brief note at the end of a letter:

Patient F.A.
My son, Frank, is also using progesterone since February.
Frank (age 15) has autism. Over the last few months he
has been less anxious and calmer. He is more outgoing in
social situations. He has been voted student of the month
for February and March. At school he is participating more,
and the teaching staff finds less prompting is necessary.
Overall, lots of nice changes.

In my view, it seems likely that eliminating most of the 40-plus vaccinations that many infants receive might also help prevent autism.

The following e-mails were sent to me by the mother of a three-year-old child with autism associated with Potocki-Lupski syndrome (PTLS) who had been essentially noncommunicative prior to treatment:

02/20/2104 (treatment started on 02/17/2014):
Ian has been great! We are all really impressed with him. He has HEAPS more energy, his speech has improved a lot suddenly, and he has been falling asleep amazingly easily and staying asleep. It is 9 p.m. now, I am ready to pass out, and he is super happy and lively and drawing and playing! We have never seen him this bright!

03/17/2014:
Anyway, I am improving and Ian is doing amazingly on the progesterone! He is really starting to talk! He is able to put more words together and is really trying to communicate. His energy and focus are way better. We are super delighted with him and cannot believe the change. It is getting some attention in the alternative health circles that I frequent.

03/24/2014:
I am going to have to really study this subject now, as Ian is doing REALLY WELL on your program! His energy is up, his speech is exploding, and he is acting so much more like a regular little boy. It is great. Even his GP is starting to get impressed; she is coming around and getting interested in this field!

POST-TRAUMATIC STRESS DISORDER

Post-traumatic stress disorder (PTSD) may also be related to excess adrenaline. PTSD is frequently diagnosed in soldiers returning from war zones. It is my feeling that most enlistees in the armed forces have large amounts of adrenaline to begin with, and this excess is probably exacerbated under the conditions of war.

PTSD is also found in trauma patients—women who have been raped, people involved in motor vehicle accidents, and so on. I suspect that many of their symptoms, such as anxiety, depression, obsessive-compulsive behavior, nervousness, and nightmares, are related to excess adrenaline.

Perhaps the most suggestive evidence of hyperadrenalism in these patients is the recent success in treating this disorder with propranolol, a powerful beta-blocker. Since the action of beta-blockers is to block the effects of adrenaline, propranolol's effectiveness with PTSD suggests that adrenaline is involved. However, propanolol is just another Band-Aid approach with a lot of side effects. Taking steps to directly lower adrenaline levels might make more sense for this condition and certainly should be worth trying.

PREMENSTRUAL DYSPHORIC DISORDER

Premenstrual dysphoric disorder (PMDD) has a tremendous impact on the quality of life of the woman who is afflicted with it, as well as the people around her. Like many other conditions discussed in this book, its cause is considered unknown.

PMDD affects about 5 percent of women who are menstruating. As with PMS, the symptoms of PMDD occur about a week before the period and generally resolve two or three days after the period starts. Although PMDD shares some characteristics with PMS, it is in a category all by itself because of the severity of the symptoms. They are bad enough to interfere with the woman's daily routine. The classic symptoms include:

- Extreme mood changes
- Depression with feelings of hopelessness
- Severe anger issues
- An underlying, pervasive anxiety
- Brain fog with difficulty focusing
- Trouble falling asleep or staying asleep
- Overwhelming fatigue
- Muscle aches and pains
- Headaches

By now, the reader probably recognizes all of these symptoms as related to adrenaline. However, PMDD has additional symptoms caused by estrogen dominance: uterine cramps, breast tenderness, fluid retention, and bloating.

Eliminating this condition begins with the clear understanding that it is strictly a hormonal problem, caused primarily by too much adrenaline and estrogen, and too little progesterone. (In spite of how it is normally treated, it is not caused by a deficiency of Prozac.) Just before her monthly period, a woman experiences a sharp drop in progesterone, which initiates menstruation. A low progesterone level leads to a rise in insulin, which, in turn, can cause hypoglycemic episodes, along with bloating, fluid retention, and weight gain. I suspect that women who have PMDD have creative type or mixed type ADHD, which makes their response to hypoglycemia more pronounced, resulting in the output of large amounts of adrenaline.

Eliminating PMDD begins with understanding it as strictly a hormonal problem.

Treatment to lower the adrenaline level, of course, is a combination of using a topical progesterone cream and following a low-glycemic meal plan. This regimen will also help to control insulin as well as block the effects of high estrogen. I received the following letter from a woman who was suffering from extreme PMDD. I present it in its entirety, despite its length, because it touches on a number of important issues, the most significant being the profound lack of knowledge about hormones among many doctors. Unfortunately, this includes many gynecologists, who are the primary specialists treating women and teenage girls.

I believe that this letter should be required reading for all doctors training to be gynecologists. Any doctor reading this who recognizes that he or she would have taken the same approach as the physicians in this letter is strongly encouraged to read my manual for healthcare practitioners: *The Platt Protocol for Hormone Balancing.*

This letter should be required reading for all doctors training to be gynecologists.

Dear Dr. Platt,

I am 33 years of age and I really do not think I will make it to 34!!! I am taking antidepressants, painkillers, and have a Mirena coil fitted. I do not have any children. I started my periods at 14 and I have suffered with severe PMS since I was 16 years old, and I really can't cope with it any more. I am sick to death of doctors not listening to me!!! I have said to them from the start that I have problems with my hormones. My own mother suffered all of her adult life with severe PMS. I am like a carbon copy of her. She had to have a hysterectomy in her early 40s to stop her PMS and has been on all sorts of HRT. She now uses estrogel, and from all I have read about "synthetic hormones" I am very worried about her. My grandmother died of breast cancer in her mid 50s, my mother is in her mid 50s!!!!!! Also my mother's aunt now has breast cancer.

I was put on a birth control pill at 15 to regulate my periods; from the onset they have been very heavy and irregular. I have since been on every contraception pill you can think of!!! Since I was 19 I have been on every antidepressant you can think of!!! I have constantly told the doctors that I am only depressed for two weeks of the month and that my problems are hormonal, but they will just not listen to me!!!

When I saw a psychologist (I had to practically beg the doctors that I wanted to see someone, as I thought I was going insane every month), she confirmed what I knew all along. I had PMDD. I then had to ask the doctors to refer me to a gynecologist.

The gynecologist gave me Provera injections, which made me worse. I felt like I was 100 years old, I have never felt so ill, so I stopped that as well. He asked if there was a possibility I could have endometriosis, how should I know! I have suffered with extremely painful periods since I can remember; I have had a very painful lower back and left shoulder since I was 23. The doctors have been aware of all of this. As the years have progressed, so has the mental and physical pain. I have been told on numerous occasions that "some people suffer painful periods, it's normal."

My gynecologist performed a laparoscopy in March this year and told me I have stage 2-3 endometriosis!!! Well, no kidding!! At the same time he fitted a Mirena coil and said this should help with the pain.

I told my gynecologist from the start that I need something for the psychological effects of PMDD as well. Yes, I am in excruciating pain every month, but what about my mental state!!! I feel like I am going insane every month. He said you do not have PMDD, you have endometriosis, which can cause mood swings!!! I suffer with a lot more than mood swings!!!

The coil has done nothing to help with the pain; if anything, it's worse. As for the PMDD, well, it's two weeks of a "living hell" for me and my close family. I become a different person; it's as though I have been possessed. My mind has been taken over and I cannot control it no matter how hard I try. I become extremely agitated, angry, nasty, bouts of uncontrollable crying, deep dark morbid thoughts, extremely depressed, suicidal thoughts, thoughts of harming others—the list is endless. And then there's the physical pain, swollen and sore breasts, bloating (I look like I'm 6 months pregnant), my hands are always swollen, I have aches and pains throughout my body, joints ache, my head aches, I have lower back and shoulder pain, pelvic pain, zero energy and motivation. I could go on!!!

I have been a guinea pig now for 18 years, trying

everything possible from contraceptive pills, injections to stop my ovaries from working, etc., and nothing has worked. I have repeatedly told the gynecologist that it is the hormones that are causing my problems, why would I want to add more of them back into my body, especially if they are synthetic. I have gained a lot of weight and the scales keep rising, even though I hardly eat a thing!!!

My gynecologist said he will perform a hysterectomy at the end of this year if I am still no better. Only a miracle could help me now, as I am not all of a sudden going to get better. While I was waiting for an appointment, I came across your book The Miracle of Bio-Identical Hormones. *I could not believe what I was reading. It confirmed my beliefs about my hormones—do my doctors have no common sense!!!*

Your book was a revelation to me: of course it's my hormones. I have known this all along, and I also knew that the amount of "synthetic" hormones they have been pumping through my body for years has made my endometriosis and PMDD so much worse.

I told my next gynecologist that I wanted to try "bio-identical hormones"—she basically laughed in my face!! She said it was all a gimmick to make money on the internet and that the patches she was going to prescribe were "bio-identical hormones" that were derived from plant extracts so that makes them bio-identical and that the molecular structure had been changed slightly!!!! (Well, it's not bio-identical, then, is it!!!) She was very patronizing. I could have had a full-blown argument with her, but to be honest I didn't have the energy and I thought, "She is my last hope"!!!

I was prescribed Estraderm MX 100; each patch contains 3 mg of estradiol!!!! From the research I have carried out, this is the worst thing I could be on!!!! I asked her if the patches would make my endometriosis worse, and she said it would be unlikely!!!! WHAT!!! Doesn't estradiol feed endometriosis??? I couldn't believe it when she said "Well, your own body produces estrogen doesn't it!!! It's the progesterone that is causing you all of your problems as this is what peaks during the last two weeks of the month when you are having problems." I could not believe what I was hearing. As you can now imagine, I do not know which way to turn.

Because of the PMDD I have never been able to keep a job for long. I am unemployed; I have been for years now. I am existing, not living. I had so many hopes and dreams which have all been taken away from me. We only have one life, and I have wasted so many years of it. All my relationships have failed, I have no friends, I have no zest for life, all I see are dark tunnels, I am a recluse, I do not go out, I really do not have a life. It's just me and the four walls. I live with my parents still, which is very hard for me. I was once a positive, bubbly, outgoing, happy person, but with each year passing I am becoming more and more negative, angry, frustrated, and extremely depressed. I am trapped within my own skin. All I want is to be free from my mind and body, and the only way I can see this happening is if I end my life. I know this may sound drastic, but I really cannot cope with the ups and downs any more and it seems the only solution.

I suppose this is a cry for help, I feel as though you are now my last chance of hope, I am desperate for help. I don't

*think I have any more tears in me to cry, and I don't have
the energy to face another dark day.
    Yours gratefully and hopefully,
    (name withheld)*

What a tragic story! This woman is clearly estrogen
dominant, as evidenced by her cramps, breast tenderness,
endometriosis, and bloating, all caused by a deficiency of
progesterone. Her doctors put her on birth control pills,
Provera, and a Mirena coil—all of which stopped her from
making progesterone. As a result, she went from a low level of
progesterone to none, which increased her symptoms related
to both estrogen dominance and adrenaline dominance. To
make matters worse, she was placed on high levels of estradiol,
the strongest estrogen, exacerbating her estrogen-induced
endometriosis.

Since few doctors are aware of the connection between
PMDD and adrenaline, her doctors could not see that
excess adrenaline was causing her mood swings, anger
issues, depression, and weight gain, as well as pains due to
fibromyalgia.

This woman has cried out for help for many years, yet
her doctors were not listening, and they failed to realize that
they did not have the knowledge to help her. Unfortunately,
this kind of story will continue until the day when patients
become angry enough to demand a more intelligent approach
from their doctors. To quote the French philosopher Voltaire:

*Doctors give drugs of which they know little,
into bodies of which they know less,
for diseases of which they know nothing at all.*

CHAPTER 7

FEN-PHEN: ANOTHER SIDE TO THE STORY

Fen-Phen—the combination of two generic weight loss drugs, fenfluramine and phentermine—was a short-lived phenomenon in medical history. At the time of its withdrawal in 1997 by the FDA, 29 million Americans were on this drug combination, and every type of medical practitioner, including primary care doctors, orthopedists, psychiatrists, and plastic surgeons, was prescribing it.

I have included Fen-Phen in this book because, in my view, no other combination of medications has lowered adrenaline and insulin levels as dramatically.

First, some background. Michael Weintraub, M.D., who is credited with combining these two weight control medications, thought that putting them together would enhance their effectiveness while reducing their side effects. His 65-page article in the May 1992 issue of *Clinical Pharmacology and Therapeutics* delineated the remarkable results of a weight loss study Weintraub had conducted using Fen-Phen.

Soon after the article appeared, a number of weight loss clinics started utilizing this drug combination and duplicated his success. The media caught on, coining the term "Fen-Phen." Almost overnight, clinics sprang up all over the country, and doctors from all specialties started prescribing it. The problem was that very few doctors really knew how to prescribe it or what the correct dosage should be.

Since phentermine and fenfluramine were generic medications—that is, they were no longer patented—no drug companies were marketing them. This eliminated the most common way that doctors learn dosing of a drug, which is from the representative of the drug company making the drug. Instead, doctors referred to the PDR (Physicians' Desk Reference), which listed the usual dosage for each medication individually—phentermine 30 mg per day and fenfluramine 20 mg three times a day—but no dosage for the combination. Having no better information, doctors simply prescribed the individual dosage for each drug—which eventually resulted in the demise of Fen-Phen.

In the meantime, A.H. Robins, the drug company that manufactured fenfluramine under the name Pondimin, came out with a new weight loss drug called Redux to replace Pondimin, which had gone off patent. Needless to say, the company wanted Fen-Phen off the market, since it could dramatically interfere with sales of Redux.

In retrospect, the decision to develop Redux never made sense. It was the same chemical as Pondimin, only stronger. And, like Pondimin, it was not very effective for weight loss when used by itself, and it had serious side effects such as pulmonary hypertension.

A.H. Robins sponsored a study conducted at the Mayo Clinic, the primary purpose of which was to eliminate Fen-Phen. They rounded up 24 women from across the United States, all on high dosages of Fen-Phen, some taking 18 times the correct dosage. Many of these women were found to have heart valve damage. As a result of this (purposely) flawed study, the FDA immediately pulled fenfluramine from the market, as well as Redux, which A.H. Robins should have anticipated. So they wound up being hoisted by their own petard.

To my knowledge, this was the only study of Fen-Phen that ever demonstrated significant heart valve damage. Between 1992 and 1997 (the year Fen-Phen was taken off the market), only five deaths were attributed to Fen-Phen. This number is minimal compared to the hundreds of thousands of deaths caused by NSAIDs, such as Vioxx and ibuprofen, or diabetic drugs such as Avandia—drugs that are still on the market or were taken off the market after many years of the FDA ignoring the number of deaths they caused.

Weintraub actually provided the correct (and safe) dosage of Fen-Phen in the epilogue to his 65-page article. In the epilogue, he comments that the dosage he used in the original study was too high, but once the study started he couldn't change the protocol. In the study he recommended a dosage of phentermine 30 mg and fenfluramine 20 mg three times a day. However, he realized after the study, started that the dosage should have been phentermine 15 mg and fenfluramine 20 mg once a day. It seems that few doctors, if any, were aware of this information.

The problem with the higher-than-necessary dosage of Fen-Phen is that while one drug, phentermine, suppressed the appetite, the other drug, fenfluramine, took away cravings. When the doses of both were too high, people stopped eating, so their metabolism halted and no weight loss occurred. The next week they would go back to their physicians and say, "Doc, I'm not losing weight," and usually the doctor prescribed an even higher dose. This scenario was sometimes repeated week after week—no wonder people got overdosed.

However, when Fen-Phen was used correctly, nothing was more effective for weight loss, and I suspect nothing ever will be. Because one drug took away the appetite and the other took away cravings, this combination allowed people to have complete control over how they ate, which contributed strongly to weight loss. In addition, I would put Fen-Phen, when used correctly, up against almost any drug on the market today in terms of safety.

When Fen-Phen was used correctly, nothing was more effective for weight loss, and I suspect nothing ever will be.

I suspect that the main reason why Fen-Phen helped bring about significant weight loss was because of fenfluramine's apparently unique ability to reduce the effect of insulin, the main hormone that creates fat from sugar and prevents the release of fat from fat cells. As long as people on Fen-Phen were eating, they were able to burn fat and lose weight.

As it turned out, Fen-Phen took away cravings not only for food but also for alcohol, cigarettes, cocaine, and heroin, usually within 24 hours. At times, I prescribed Fen-Phen just to get a patient off cigarettes—which was 100 percent successful—and the weight gain that commonly occurs after people stop smoking never happened.

Used together, the combination of phentermine and fenfluramine lowered blood pressure, eliminated migraine headaches, and, quite remarkably, got rid of asthma, depression, and ADHD. It also helped diabetics to get off their medications. In fact, I found Fen-Phen more successful in getting rid of these conditions than any other medication on the market. Fen-Phen appears to have helped prevent the effects of not only insulin but also of adrenaline. I suspect that because insulin was controlled, there was less hypoglycemia, which meant that less adrenaline was released to raise the sugar level. This drop in adrenaline helped to eliminate high blood pressure and ADHD. Individually, phentermine or fenfluramine could elevate blood pressure. However, the combination actually lowered it.

Sadly, the FDA's primary function often appears to be protecting drug companies rather than benefiting consumers. Fen-Phen was pulled from the market based on a study of only 24 women who were on extremely high doses of the medications—clearly an invalid study. In fact, extremely few deaths have been attributed to this drug combination, and very few side effects occurred when the correct dose was used.

Compare this to Chantix, a drug on the market since 2006 to aid in smoking cessation, which has been found to increase the risk of a heart attack or stroke by 72 percent. In other words, one in twenty-eight users will develop this problem. Chantix also causes erratic behavior and depression, along with suicidal thoughts. In 2009, Chantix received a black box warning concerning these issues, and as of 2011, more than 150 suicides had been attributed to this drug. Yet it is still on the market.

Fen-Phen was eliminated from the market because of heart concerns, yet I do not know of any drug combination that has actually been more beneficial for the heart.

Fen-Phen was eliminated from the market because of heart concerns, yet I do not know of any drug combination that has actually been more beneficial for the heart. Fen-Phen helped people get off cigarettes, lowered blood pressure, helped to eliminate diabetes, reduced stress, and was the most successful non-surgical treatment ever for losing excess weight.

I researched this drug combination for six months before I started using it with patients. The first patient I put on it lost 100 pounds in three months with only minor changes his eating habits.

In this era of epidemic obesity, it might be worthwhile for the medical community to reassess the positive aspects of Fen-Phen. This would require a reevaluation of its benefits, an honest reassessment of its safety and efficacy, and FDA reapproval.

This kind of reapproval of a drug happened not too long ago for a hypnotic medication called thalidomide. In the 1950s and 1960s, this drug had been prescribed as a sleeping aid for pregnant women, which unfortunately resulted in a significant number of congenital birth defects, and it was taken off the market. Subsequently, it was found to have unique qualities that allowed its reemergence as an anti-rejection drug used with transplant patients.

If Fen-Phen is ever reintroduced, steps must be taken to ensure correct dosing. Perhaps a limited study could be funded by the NIH, focusing on treatment of the morbidly obese. I doubt if drug companies would be interested in doing these studies, since phentermine and fenfluramine are not patentable.

Perhaps it is time for the medical community to accept the fact that the current recommendations for controlling weight are not working. Surgery should not be the answer.

Since obesity is now considered a disease rather than an eating problem, the idea of using medications to treat it might also be more acceptable. If a weight loss medication can also eliminate hypertension, asthma, migraine headaches, substance addictions, ADHD, and depression, so much the better.

Interestingly, bio-identical progesterone cream provides many of the same clinical results as Fen-Phen because of its effect on insulin and adrenaline. It also helps with weight loss, though the effect is not as profound as with Fen-Phen.

CHAPTER 8

ADRENAL FATIGUE— OR IS IT?

A drenal fatigue is a diagnosis used mostly in alternative medicine, usually among naturopathic physicians. The diagnosis is based on the theory that the adrenal gland, if underfunctioning, can fail to produce sufficient quantities of cortisol. Treatment often involves prescribing cortisol in addition to addressing diet, timing of eating, and amount of rest.

I have two concerns about this diagnosis and its treatment. First, adrenal fatigue may actually be adrenaline dominance, a condition of adrenal overfunctioning rather than underfunctioning. Second, prescribing cortisol for a condition possibly already associated with a high cortisol level may have unintended consequences. Cortisol, if given inappropriately, can produce unwanted weight gain by raising sugar and insulin levels. It can also cause osteoporosis, cataracts, stomach ulcers, muscle wasting, and brain damage.

Naturopathic physician James Wilson, in his book, *Adrenal Fatigue: The 21st Century Stress Syndrome*,* published in 2001, gives a list of symptoms suggesting adrenal fatigue. These include:

---

* J.L.Wilson, *Adrenal Fatigue: The 21st Century Stress Syndrome* (Petaluma, CA: Smart Publications, 2001), pp. 27–45.

- Fatigue unrelieved by sleep
- Difficulty falling asleep and staying asleep
- Decreased ability to handle stress
- Depression
- Increased PMS in women
- Increased symptoms when meals are skipped
- Problems focusing, with memory lapses
- Decreased tolerance, easily irritated
- Low energy between 3 and 4 p.m.
- Difficulty staying on task
- Being easily startled, which causes palpitations
- Anxiety attacks
- Hypoglycemia
- Weight gain

As we have seen in this book, excess adrenaline can cause or contribute to every one of these symptoms.

So is adrenal fatigue a condition related to too little cortisol or too much adrenaline? The distinction is important, since the treatments for the two conditions differ.

So is adrenal fatigue a condition related to too little cortisol or too much adrenaline? The distinction is important, since the treatments for the two conditions differ. Usually, symptoms related to excess adrenaline can be largely relieved within 24 hours. Problems related to adrenal fatigue are more complex, since adrenal insufficiency can take months to correct.

I suspect that one of the sources of confusion between adrenaline dominance and adrenal fatigue is that a low level of salivary cortisol is often considered an indicator of adrenal fatigue. However, I have observed that patients with low cortisol levels in saliva often have high cortisol levels in the blood. An elevated cortisol in a morning blood sample almost always goes along with high adrenaline. In fact, I consider a high morning cortisol blood level to be the best indicator of high adrenaline. (In my view, any cortisol level greater than 11.5 might actually be considered elevated.)

I believe that this significant discrepancy between high cortisol levels in the blood versus low levels in the saliva is related to the tendency of adrenaline to constrict blood vessels. For example, the most common cause of cold hands and cold feet is excess adrenaline, not low thyroid. Vasoconstriction of blood vessels in the eye can cause glaucoma (which is often treated with beta-blocker eye drops), and vasoconstriction of the vestibular artery in the neck can cause tinnitus in the ears. Similarly, vasoconstriction of salivary gland blood vessels could possibly restrict blood flow to that area, resulting in low cortisol levels in the salivary glands themselves (as well as a dry mouth, which is commonly found in people with anxiety).

It might make more sense to treat patients initially as if they have adrenaline dominance.

For these reasons, it might make more sense to treat patients initially as if they have adrenaline dominance, rather than starting them on cortisol, a powerful hormone that they may not need. The fact that excess adrenaline responds so quickly to the protocol presented in this book can be used as a diagnostic tool. If the patient's symptoms are caused by adrenaline dominance, the symptoms should disappear or at least improve within 24 hours. If the symptoms do not improve within 24 hours, then the possibility of adrenal fatigue can be considered.

Cortef, the drug most commonly used to treat adrenal fatigue, raises the cortisol level. Patients often feel better after they have started on Cortef. This may be because Cortef also raises the blood sugar level, which can decrease the body's need to put out adrenaline. It can also act as an antidepressant. Thus Cortef can appear to be helping, whereas it may actually be making things worse.

A word of caution: If a morning blood cortisol test shows that the patient's cortisol level is below normal, and if the person's DHEA-S (dehydroepiandrosterone-sulfate, a hormone produced by the adrenal gland) level is also extremely low, the patient should probably be referred to an endocrinologist for treatment of possible Addison's disease—a true condition of "adrenal fatigue."

CHAPTER 9 | MANAGING EXCESS ADRENALINE

This chapter discusses the specifics of the treatment protocol for managing excess adrenaline. This treatment can bring about improvement of many of the conditions caused by adrenaline dominance fairly quickly, often within 24 hours. The two main aspects of the protocol—using progesterone cream and following a properly balanced diet—are discussed separately. (A recommended eating plan is provided in the appendix.) Both are vital to lowering adrenaline, though they play different roles. Progesterone lowers adrenaline indirectly through its effect on insulin. The only thing that directly lowers adrenaline is giving the brain a steady supply of the right fuel so the body doesn't continue to release adrenaline. This is accomplished through diet.

This treatment can bring about improvement of many of the conditions caused by adrenaline dominance fairly quickly, often within 24 hours.

Because of the damage that can occur from prolonged imbalance of neurotransmitters in the brain, this chapter also includes a section on recommended supplements to improve brain health. The final section comments on diet and supplements for children with ADHD and autism.

DIETARY TREATMENT: A MEAL PLAN

The importance of diet in treating hyperadrenalism cannot be underestimated. It represents 70 percent of the successful approach to lowering adrenaline and is essential in addressing all of the conditions mentioned in this book: the "good," the "bad," and the "ugly" manifestations of excess adrenaline. In my view, we can assume that everyone who has one or more of the "bad" or "ugly" conditions caused by adrenaline dominance also has one of its "good" aspects: typical type, creative type, or mixed type ADHD.

The meal plan for reducing adrenaline is designed around the principle of providing a steady supply of fuel for the body and especially for the brain. It relies on the glycemic index, which rates foods according to how quickly and how high they raise the level of glucose in the blood, and, consequently, the level of insulin. A useful version of the glycemic index is available in appendix B.

The meal plan for reducing adrenaline is designed around the principle of providing a steady supply of fuel for the body and especially for the brain.

A food high on the glycemic index is digested quickly and releases sugars into the bloodstream rapidly, which means it keeps the blood sugar yo-yoing due to alternating high sugar–high insulin levels. Examples of high-glycemic foods are refined sugar, refined grains or flours, many fruits, and all the products made with these foods.

Foods ranked low on the glycemic index are digested more slowly and release sugars more gradually, so a diet that focuses on low-glycemic foods prevents the yo-yo effect and thereby helps to control adrenaline. Low-glycemic foods include whole grains and legumes, vegetables, some fruits, and unprocessed foods. In addition, the meal plan for reducing adrenaline includes healthy fats, good protein, and sufficient water. I recommend including extra virgin coconut oil in the diet. Traditional thinking has always been that sugar, in the form of glucose, is the only fuel the brain requires. Recently, however, it has been discovered that ketone bodies might be an even more potent source of fuel for the brain. Ketone bodies are formed from medium-chain triglycerides (MCTs), which are found in coconut oil and palm oil. They are important for reducing insulin resistance in the brain (type III diabetes), and may help to prevent, and in some cases greatly alleviate, Alzheimer's disease.

The importance of avoiding high-glycemic carbohydrates to control excess adrenaline is well illustrated by revisiting the story of Jose, the nine-year-old boy with typical type ADHD who we saw in chapter 4. It was Jose's mother who brought him to me for care and who applied the progesterone cream that helped him so much. Jose's father did not believe that eating correctly was a factor in his son's improvement.

One morning he took Jose to the International House of Pancakes. Jose ordered pancakes and waffles and smothered them in syrup. Shortly thereafter, he jumped up and started throwing plates onto the floor from adjoining tables. He found the Coca-Cola dispenser and started wolfing down sodas. He began yelling and screaming; the police came and ended up detaining him overnight. The father learned firsthand that

Jose could not eat or drink refined sugar without stimulating the release of large amounts of adrenaline.

The full meal plan designed for people with excess adrenaline is available in appendix A. The logical nutritional advice it provides can benefit anyone, including people trying to lose weight.

While *what* one eats is important for managing excess adrenaline, *when* one eats is equally important. A person with any type of ADHD should ideally eat five small meals spaced every three hours throughout the day.

For people with creative type ADHD, this timing is especially critical. They need to eat often because their brains are more active. As we have seen, the brain uses more fuel than any other area in the body, and the creative brain requires a lot more fuel than a normal brain. Because of this, people with creative brains are the ones who get shaky or irritable if they go too long without eating. This, of course, is an adrenaline effect. So it's important for them to eat frequently, every three or four hours. However, anyone with any type of ADHD requires fuel for the brain. The safest and most logical approach for all people with ADHD, then, is to eat a small low-glycemic carbohydrate meal about every three hours.

For people with creative type ADHD, this timing is especially critical. They need to eat often because their brains are more active.

For all people with adrenaline dominance conditions, the importance of eating breakfast has to be stressed. And breakfast needs to be a balanced meal of protein and low-glycemic carbohydrates. This may be a challenge at first, since excess adrenaline can take away the appetite, so people with excess adrenaline conditions may be used to skipping breakfast. But if lunch is their first meal, it means the brain and muscles have gone without fuel for at least 16 hours. As a result, these people are most likely living on adrenaline, that is, they are caught in the insulin-sugar-adrenaline cycle that keeps their adrenaline level high. However, if they follow the protocols outlined here, their adrenaline levels will be significantly lower at night, and their appetite for breakfast will return.

The brain uses more fuel than any other area in the body, and the creative brain requires a lot more fuel than a normal brain.

For some people, it is also important to eat a low-glycemic snack just before bedtime so the brain doesn't run out of fuel during the night. A bedtime snack is recommended if any of the following symptoms are occurring at night: tossing and turning, restless leg syndrome, teeth grinding, hot flashes, awakening through the night, or nighttime urination.

Those with mixed type ADHD—showing characteristics of both types—need to observe the meal timing for creative type ADHD, since their brains also use large amounts of fuel.

HORMONAL TREATMENT: PROGESTERONE

Progesterone cream, used correctly, is vital to controlling excess adrenaline; it represents 30 percent of achieving success with the protocol. Progesterone cream is available by prescription in various strengths from a compounding pharmacy, or it can be obtained as an over-the-counter (OTC) preparation. The object is to obtain a cream that is bio-identical, which means it is identical in molecular structure to the progesterone produced by both men and women. The cream is made from a natural source, either yam or soy. If an OTC label says "wild yam extract" and does not also say "USP progesterone," it is best to avoid that cream, since the body has no way of converting yam extract into progesterone.

Bio-identical progesterone cream is extremely safe. I have never heard of anyone overdosing on progesterone in this form. Some people have an allergy to soy-based products; people with this allergy may develop a rash where a soy-based bio-identical cream is applied.

Bio-identical progesterone cream is extremely safe. I have never heard of anyone overdosing on progesterone in this form.

Application: How Much, When, and Where

The initial dosage I recommend is 50 mg, three times a day, applied one to three minutes before breakfast, lunch, and dinner. Later on, doses can be adjusted downward as the symptoms lessen.

The best way to determine if the dose is correct is to assess how the person is feeling. He or she should no longer be getting hypoglycemic (sleepy) between 3 and 4 p.m. or while in a car or after eating. The person may have started to lose weight. If excess adrenaline was a concern, the person should be more relaxed, sleeping better, focusing better, and less irritable. Premenopausal women should experience a marked reduction in PMS, cramps, breast tenderness, and so on. Migraine headaches and asthma should be gone.

The best way to determine if the dose is correct is to assess how the person is feeling.

If the person is still getting sleepy in the afternoon, he or she may not be applying the cream at the right times. For controlling insulin, timing can be critical. The body releases insulin as soon as food hits the tongue, so the progesterone must be in the bloodstream before eating. Since progesterone is short-lived in the blood stream, I recommend applying the progesterone cream one to three minutes before a meal. The body puts out the most insulin in the afternoon, so the progesterone cream application just before lunch is possibly the most important of the day.

For people who have creative type ADHD and have trouble staying asleep through the night, eating a snack of low-glycemic carbohydrates just before going to bed is important. Progesterone cream should be applied one to three minutes before this bedtime snack.

Perhaps the easiest site for applying the cream is the inner forearm. After the cream is applied, the two forearms should be rubbed together so the cream can be absorbed over a wide surface area. For people who suffer from tinnitus (ringing in the ear) or who get traction (tension) headaches, I recommend placing the cream on the back of the neck. Someone with a migraine headache may find that the headache is gone three to four minutes after applying the cream to the forearms and forehead.

Avoid placing the cream over fatty areas, such as the abdomen or inner thighs. The forearms, the back of the neck, the cheeks, and the upper chest are better because in those areas the skin is thin and there is a good blood supply.

Eventually, some time after applying the cream, the level of progesterone in the brain will be 20 times higher than anywhere else. This affinity for brain tissue explains why progesterone has such a marked effect on neurotransmitters in the brain, and why it is so effective at reducing swelling in traumatic brain injuries. Perhaps football players, who are subject to head injuries, should be using it routinely.

Notably, the incredibly high levels of progesterone that occur in the second and third trimesters during pregnancy help the fetal brain to develop. I am hoping that some day it will occur to neonatologists that they should be providing bio-identical progesterone to premature infants.

Special Considerations When Using Progesterone

For the most part, progesterone cream is extremely well tolerated. However, progesterone can significantly affect how the body functions, and people tend to react to hormones differently, so some people may experience side effects from progesterone. In my experience, if side effects occur, they are usually temporary. A major benefit of bio-identical creams is that it is easy to titrate the dose or change the area of application and thus reduce or avoid side effects. Side effects may include:

- Headaches and/or dizziness (extremely rare)
- Acne (uncommon)
- Sleepiness (only when used orally)
- Menstrual spotting or heavier periods
- Nipple tenderness in women

In most cases, progesterone cream actually eliminates the first three side effects listed. Women with migraine headaches secondary to estrogen may find that their headache disappears within minutes after using progesterone. In the rare cases where headaches do occur as a side effect of progesterone, I recommend either temporarily reducing the dose or applying the cream on the inner ankle, which allows the progesterone to attach to many receptor sites as it moves through the bloodstream before reaching the head.

Acne, which can be triggered by elevated testosterone, often improves with progesterone because the progesterone can lead to a decrease in testosterone production in women who overproduce it. This is often seen in cases of polycystic ovarian syndrome (PCOS). However, progesterone can also downregulate into other hormones including testosterone, and thus can cause acne. If this is the case, I would decrease the dose or ask the patient to apply it at her ankle. This side effect should eventually disappear. If the problem persists, obtaining a prescription for spironolactone, 25–50 mg/day, may be helpful. This drug can block the production of testosterone.

Sleepiness or fatigue is rare as a side effect of progesterone cream, but it is common with any type of oral progesterone, including Prometrium, progesterone troches, and drops placed under the tongue. This is because any form of oral progesterone goes directly to the liver, where it converts into allopregnanolone, which does cause fatigue. This is why Prometrium is always prescribed at bedtime. With progesterone in cream form, on the other hand, fatigue from hypoglycemia is usually eliminated, since progesterone controls insulin.

Because progesterone can block adrenaline, a person starting on progesterone cream may experience a noticeable loss of energy, especially if he or she has been "living on adrenaline" (for example, those with a type A personality). If thyroid levels are on the lower side of normal, excess adrenaline can sometimes mask the fatigue typically associated with subclinical hypothyroidism. In this case, the person, when first starting progesterone cream, can experience significant fatigue, which can be eliminated by adding thyroid medication.

In some people, the sudden drop in adrenaline has a dramatic effect on the body comparable to the sudden withdrawal from a psychoactive medication, and can cause unpleasant side effects, such as uncontrollable crying. I have seen this most often in people whose level of adrenaline—the rage and anger hormone—was very high. The crying jag is most likely an expression of relief and is a temporary phenomenon.

Rarely, some people show an increase in adrenaline-like symptoms such as palpitations, nervousness, and trouble sleeping. The cause for this is unclear. It could be the body responding to the sudden drop in adrenaline by increasing the production of this hormone. Or it could be related to progesterone blocking the insulin receptor sites of brain cells, which in effect lowers the sugar level inside the brain cells, causing the release of adrenaline to raise the sugar level. In these cases, I recommend reducing the dose of progesterone temporarily, allowing the body to acclimate to it more slowly, and then gradually increasing the dose to an effective level.

If menstrual spotting occurs when a woman starts using progesterone cream, or if the menstrual flow is heavier, it is often because the progesterone is bringing about healing of the uterus. These effects usually go away after several months. In some cases, progesterone can initially downregulate into estradiol (one of the three forms of estrogen), in which case the progesterone dose may actually need to be increased to balance the increase in estrogen. This side effect is more commonly seen when using a low dose (2%) over-the-counter progesterone cream.

Women trying to conceive may want to replicate the hormonal pattern of the normal menstrual cycle, which means not using the progesterone cream from day one to day ten of their cycle.

Because there are many progesterone receptor sites around the nipples, some women may experience tenderness in this area when first starting on progesterone cream. In these cases, the dose can be cut in half until the discomfort disappears and then returned to full dose.

Progesterone causes apoptosis (death) of breast cancer cells. For this reason, I consider progesterone beneficial for women who have or have had breast cancer that is progesterone receptor site positive. Most oncologists would probably disagree. However, their knowledge of progesterone is usually limited to synthetic progestins, such as Provera (medroxyprogesterone), which can cause the same side effects as estrogen: breast cancer, blood clots, and weight gain. Bio-identical progesterone, which behaves in the body quite differently from synthetic progestins, has none of these side effects.

Remarkably, the State of California has, for some reason, decided that bio-identical progesterone causes cancer. This is in spite of the fact that in the 70 years of its existence it has never been demonstrated to cause cancer. Ironically, estrogen is a known cancer-causing chemical, yet it is injected into animals to fatten them (even though injecting a carcinogenic substance into an animal for this purpose is illegal).

SUPPLEMENTS FOR BRAIN HEALTH

All the hormones discussed in this book—adrenaline, progesterone, cortisol, and insulin—significantly influence brain activity. They have a strong effect on neurotransmitters in the brain, such as serotonin, GABA, dopamine, and acetylcholine. Neurotransmitters act as chemical messengers and are responsible for how neurons (brain cells) communicate with one another. They influence memory, mood, alertness, and thinking. Every single external stimulus perceived through touch, smell, vision, taste, or hearing results in the release of neurotransmitters.

All the hormones discussed in this book— adrenaline, progesterone, cortisol, and insulin—have a strong effect on neurotransmitters, which are responsible for how brain cells communicate with one another.

Brain cell function is affected not only by these chemical messengers but also by the membranes surrounding the brain cells. The cell membrane acts as a barrier, or gateway, that prevents certain harmful substances from entering the cell and, at the same time, allows necessary compounds inside.

As is true everywhere else in the body, the chemical processes involved in brain function tend to run more smoothly when things are in balance. For a thorough explanation of this important subject, I highly recommend the book *The UltraMind Solution* by Mark Hyman, M.D., published in 2008. Dr. Hyman explains that low levels of dopamine are associated with problems of focusing and decreased energy.

Low dopamine levels have been noted in people with ADHD and agitated depression—an observation that provides a rationale for treating these conditions with drugs like Ritalin, which is similar to adrenaline.

Needless to say, I disagree with this approach, since, in my view, these people already have too much adrenaline, which may be suppressing their production of dopamine. If this is the case, it would be better to lower the adrenaline level in order to raise the dopamine level and improve the patient's focus.

Dr. Hyman also points out that some people may be dopamine resistant. This is a problem that can be reversed through nutrition and vitamin supplementation.

Providing metabolic support for the brain involves a combination of correct nutritional supplementation for brain cells and correct amino acid intervention to help balance neurotransmitters. A complete discussion of the nutritional requirements of the brain is beyond the scope of this book. However, the following sections discuss the key nutrients needed to support brain function and provide some fundamental recommendations to help ensure a healthy brain.

FATS

Neurons require four essential fats for their cell membranes to function: DHA, EPA, phosphatidylcholine, and phosphatidylserine. "Essential" in this context means that the body cannot manufacture these substances; they must be obtained through diet or supplements. These fats, or fatty acids, are necessary for the formation of acetylcholine, a neurotransmitter that is important for our cognitive (learning) abilities as well as memory. Low levels of DHA and the other essential fatty acids in the brain are associated with a decline in thinking capacity as well as the development of Alzheimer's disease.

DHA and EPA can be obtained by eating fish or taking fish oil. The other two are best obtained as supplements:

a) Phosphatidylserine—about 300 mg per day

b) Phosphatidylcholine—best taken in the form of

L-alpha glycerylphosphorylcholine (alpha-GPC),
up to 1200 mg per day in divided doses

Another useful fat for brain cell health is coconut oil. Until recently, sugar, in the form of glucose, was regarded as the only source of fuel for the brain. It is now known that brain cells also use ketone bodies for energy. In fact, D-betahydroxybutyrate (DBH), the primary ketone body that replaces sugar for energy, is called a "brain superfuel." DBH is actually a better fuel for the brain than sugar. It acts as an antioxidant to reduce free radical damage, and it also increases oxygen levels in brain cells. The best source for DBH is from ketone bodies obtained from the metabolism of medium-chain triglycerides (MCTs) derived from extra virgin coconut oil.

Coconut oil benefits the brain in another way, as well. A recent finding is that some people have insulin resistance limited to the brain cells only—a condition called type III diabetes that is regarded as a major cause of Alzheimer's. Indeed, it is not hard to imagine that high levels of insulin can damage brain tissue similar to the way insulin causes neuropathies in the lower extremities. Most remarkably, DBH has been shown to counteract insulin resistance in the brain.

Coconut oil can be used in various ways in the diet. It can be added to a smoothie, used to cook eggs, or combined with vinegar as a salad dressing. The recommended dose is 1 to 1½ tablespoons of coconut oil per day. The dose for treating Alzheimer's is 3½ tablespoons per day.

PROTEINS

Neurotransmitters are made up of amino acids, which explains why eating protein at each meal is so important. However, supplementation with certain amino acids can sometimes be helpful, for instance, when the patient is dealing with depression or anxiety, in which case the aim would be to increase the serotonin level. Antidepressant drugs such as Prozac and Zoloft do this by inhibiting the reuptake of serotonin.

Serotonin is the neurotransmitter that helps to make us less anxious and less depressed and also helps with sleep. Foods that increase serotonin include dates, papayas, and bananas. Foods that lower serotonin include breads, especially whole wheat and rye.

The most common amino acid supplement used to raise the serotonin level is 5-hydroxytryptophan, or 5-HTP, the immediate precursor to serotonin. The dosage is 50–150 mg in the afternoon and at bedtime.

Note, however, that in order to convert 5-HTP into serotonin, the body must have sufficient levels of vitamin B6, folic acid, vitamin C, and magnesium.

Four other supplements are also useful in controlling anxiety and depression, and taking any one of them is an alternative to taking 5-HTP. They are:

Ashwagandha—200 mg per day

Holy basil—500 mg twice a day

Passion flower—100 mg per day

L-theanine—400 mg per day

GABA, or gamma-aminobutyric acid, is the major inhibitory neurotransmitter in the brain. It is produced directly in the brain from glutamate, using a form of vitamin B6 known as pyridoxal-5-phosphate. A higher level of GABA is associated with reduced anxiety and increased relaxation. GABA can be supplemented in the dosage of 500 mg twice a day. Prometrium, a form of oral progesterone mentioned earlier, causes sedation and drowsiness through its effect on GABA.

Excitogens are amino acids that act as neurotransmitters, but in an adverse way. In large amounts they can actually lead to the death of brain cells. To avoid excitogen damage to brain cells, it is wise to limit or eliminate the use of MSG (monosodium glutamate) in the diet, as well as aspartame (a sweetener found in diet drinks under the name of NutraSweet, and on the tables of many restaurants in packets of Equal).

OTHER NECESSARY NUTRIENTS

The following additional nutrients for the brain are listed in random order without any relationship to their level of importance.

Vitamin C – Vitamin C has no known level of toxicity—in other words, it's not possible to take too much—and it easily crosses the blood-brain barrier to get into the brain. Once in the brain, it helps to neutralize toxic substances, such as high levels of iron, copper, aluminum, lead, and mercury. It slows the progression of plaque development in the arteries of the brain by reducing inflammation, much as it does in the coronary arteries. I recommend using a liposomal form of this vitamin at a dose of 1000 mg. In this form of vitamin C, 1000 mg is equivalent to 8000 mg because it does not get oxidized.

Glutathione – The powerful antioxidant glutathione (GSH) is also extremely useful for detoxifying the brain of heavy metals. It is the brain's primary defense against the damaging effects of free radicals. Just about every serious brain condition—this includes Parkinson's, Alzheimer's, strokes, Huntington's, and traumatic brain injuries—is associated with low levels of GSH. Glutathione is manufactured in the body from precursor amino acids plus other substances. Supplementation is limited because the acid in the stomach destroys it. However, there is an acetylated form (acetyl-glutathione) that is supposed to be amenable to oral administration. A liposomal preparation, which protects the GSH from being degraded in the stomach, is also available.

Two other possibilities are a skin patch and intravenous administration. The latter should be mandatory for the serious brain conditions mentioned in the first paragraph.

Alpha lipoic acid – Alpha lipoic acid is an effective metal chelator for not only the brain but also the liver. It is helpful for Alzheimer's as well as other dementias. It bolsters intracellular GSH and readily crosses the blood-brain barrier into the brain. Used in conjunction with vitamin E, which also readily crosses into the brain, it has been shown to prevent damage from a stroke. The recommended dosage is 300 mg twice a day.

Curcumin – Curcumin, a compound found in turmeric, has been shown to restore memory and insulin receptors in the cerebral cortex. It also restores decreased GSH levels. In combination with DHA, it has been shown to improve Alzheimer's dementia. Some studies indicate that it helps to clear the amyloid plaques found in the brains of patients with Alzheimer's. Recommended dosage: 500 mg twice a day.

Vitamin D3 – Vitamin D3 is necessary for normal brain development. Low levels of this vitamin have been linked to depression and Alzheimer's. Low levels during pregnancy have been linked to the development of autism in the child. There are vitamin D3 receptors on just about every cell in the body. The recommended dosage issued by the Institute of Medicine (400 IU per day) is too low. A more logical dosage is 10,000 IU per day. Vitamin D3 is not a fat-soluble vitamin; it is a prohormone and therefore does not benefit from the presence of an oil. So it is best to avoid taking vitamin D3 in gel caps, since the oil in them impairs absorption to some extent.

Vitamin K2, in the form of MK-7, should always be taken along with vitamin D3 to prevent the possibility of vitamin D putting calcium into blood vessels. In fact, vitamin K2 might even pull calcium out of blood vessels. The recommended dosage of MK-7 is 180 mcg per day.

Resveratrol – Resveratrol has been shown to reduce amyloid plaque formation in brain cells, suggesting that it may benefit patients with Alzheimer's. Recommended dosage: 300–500 mg per day. A lower dose would suffice if it is combined with pterostilbene.

Magnesium – Magnesium is an anti-stress supplement, useful for problems related to anxiety, ADHD, insomnia, and autism. Recommended dosage: 1000 mg per day (reduce dose if diarrhea occurs).

Selenium – Selenium is a very valuable mineral in the body. Mostly known for its anticancer effects, it also helps the body to synthesize GSH, utilize essential fatty acids, and produce thyroid hormones. Recommended dosage: 200 mcg per day.

Zinc – Zinc is an important mineral for the immune system and for controlling inflammation in the body and the brain. It helps DNA to function, which is fundamental to how the body operates. It helps with digestion and preventing food allergies as well as eliminating heavy metals and preventing depression. Recommended dosage: 50 mg per day.

B vitamins – B vitamins are utilized in thousands of chemical reactions throughout the body, so their importance should not be underestimated. Each one is important for the brain in some way. The three most important for the brain are:

> **Vitamin B12** – in the form of methylcobalamin. Recommended dosage: 1000–5000 mcg per day.
>
> **Folic acid** – in the form of l-methylfolate. Recommended dosage: at least 800 mcg per day.
>
> **Vitamin B6** – in the form of pyridoxal-5-phosphate. Recommended dosage: 50 mg per day.

Berberine – Berberine is not a well-known supplement, but I suspect it will be gaining popularity. Traditionally, it has been used to improve utilization of glucose and help with cholesterol metabolism in diabetic patients. However, it is now on the list of supplements to help prevent Alzheimer's. It seems to help prevent type III diabetes, which is insulin resistance in the brain. I recommend that all people with diabetes consider taking this supplement, as they are at increased risk of developing Alzheimer's. Recommended dosage: 1000 mg per day.

DIET AND SUPPLEMENTS FOR CHILDREN WITH ADHD OR AUTISM

Supplement recommendations for children with ADHD or autism deserve special mention in this book. The brains of children with ADHD or autism are extremely active. It is not hard to surmise that excess adrenaline, insulin, and cortisol could be causing irregularities in their neurotransmitters and damage to their neurons.

I am very aware of the difficulty parents often have trying to provide nutritional support for these children. All I can suggest is: do the best you can. Green vegetables are the perfect form of sugar for children's brains. If these can be provided in the form of a green smoothie, a number of supplements can also be added to the mixture by opening up capsules or using supplements in liquid form.

At minimum, I would recommend daily: vitamin D3 in a dose of at least 5000 IU; a B complex that includes B12 (500 mcg), folic acid (800 mcg), and B6 (10 mg) in the forms mentioned earlier; and some fish oil.

For children with autism, I would recommend a diet very high in green vegetables along with some form of digestive enzymes so that they can metabolize the carbohydrates to provide fuel for their brains. Every meal should include protein along with low-glycemic carbohydrates. I would also recommend about three tablespoons of coconut oil per day, along with the supplements listed in the prior paragraph. Non-communicative autistic children may have a food allergy to gluten or casein (found in milk products); it has been reported that removing these allergens from their diet often gets them to start talking.

AFTERWORD	# THOUGHTS ON THE STANDARD OF CARE

This chapter may appear to have nothing to do with adrenaline dominance. However, I am including it because many of the ideas in this book are nontraditional and so might be considered outside the "standard of care." The standard of care is defined as the approach that a "prudent" doctor would take to assess and deal with a particular medical situation. It is a legal definition, not a medical definition.

All new ideas in medicine arise outside the standard of care. For example, in 1981, two doctors, Barry Marshall and Robin Warren, proposed that peptic ulcer disease was caused by the bacterium *H. pylori*, rather than from too much acid. They were ridiculed and attacked by the traditionalists of medicine for treating their patients with antibiotics. Twenty-four years later, in 2005, they were awarded the Nobel Prize in Medicine for their idea.

The point is that a "prudent" doctor is often unaware of changes occurring in medicine and is often resistant to change. Should these doctors be the ones responsible for determining the standard of care? At the end of the nineteenth century, Semmelweiss and Lister were destroyed by their medical peers for suggesting that doctors should wash their hands prior to surgery and between child deliveries. As we are all aware, washing hands is now considered fundamental to good medicine.

Enforcing the existing standard of care runs the risk of impeding progress in medicine. In California, my home state, the medical review board has lost sight of its original mission, which was to protect the consumers of California from harmful medical practices. It has become a punishment agency, often going after doctors whose ideas may be considered outside the standard of care, even though they have not harmed any patients. It is a system that rewards ignorance and punishes new ways of thinking.

Regrettably, going outside the standard of care can make a practitioner vulnerable to losing his or her license, even when he or she has caused no harm. With regard to my own situation, the California medical board placed me on five years' probation, essentially for failing to do a pelvic exam on a woman I was treating for stress incontinence. At the time I saw her, she was receiving annual pelvic exams from both her internist and gynecologist and was not in need of another. To address the stress incontinence, I had the patient utilize bio-identical testosterone cream intravaginally, along with doing Kegel exercises to build up the periurethral muscles to eliminate the incontinence.

In more than 90 percent of cases, testosterone cream plus Kegel exercises eliminates stress incontinence in three to six days. However, the "standard of care" is to prescribe a drug such as Detrol or Ditropan, which is rarely effective. Many women with this condition wind up having unsuccessful surgeries, which are also within the standard of care. And some women have vaginal meshes inserted, which are now a source of multiple lawsuits, and yet are still within the standard of care. Since the experts that the medical review board called in were in the "prudent doctor" category, I wound up being accused of multiple departures from the standard of care because of these doctors' profound lack of knowledge.

One of the stipulations of my five-year probation was to take a clinical evaluation course called PACE at the University of California San Diego. It included computerized testing, which I passed, plus a clinical evaluation by doctors—which I failed. Those doctors felt that my ideas of practicing medicine, which are delineated here as well as in my other books, *The Miracle of Bio-Identical Hormones* and *The Platt Protocol for Hormone Balancing*, were so dangerous that I should not be practicing medicine.

The doctors involved with PACE seem to have lost the ability to think or reason. If information is not provided by a drug company, they feel it cannot be true. The head of this questionable program wrote a scathing evaluation of me, even though he never spoke to me. In a newspaper interview, he indicated that he was against alternative medicine. As a result of this clearly bigoted assessment by PACE, my license was suspended.

In 40 years of practice, not a single patient of mine has ever complained to the review board that I harmed them. In spite of this, the assigned deputy attorney general pursued me for years, attempting to manufacture as much evidence as she could in order to destroy me. Relying on the clinical incompetence of the medical board's "experts," she was able to manufacture multiple allegations against me based on mistruths and ignorance. Over one hundred letters expressing support for me were sent to the board by my patients. Some of these letters are included in this book. When some of my patients called the board to support me, they were told that if they had nothing negative to say, the board was not interested. The "investigation" was clearly one-sided and a sham. I was told that none of the letters submitted in support of me were read, although there was apparently an exception. A physician from Washington State who spent a day with me in my office after I helped him eliminate his daughter's postpartum depression wrote a letter on my behalf to the California board, saying that the day he spent with me was a highlight of his medical career. I suspect they read his letter because he was a doctor. In response, the California medical board contacted the board in Washington, who went after this doctor in the same manner the California board pursued me.

The California board, as part of their strategy with me, organized a sting operation and had me arrested for talking to their undercover agent while my license was suspended. The charges were dropped several months later by a district attorney's office in Riverside County. However, under pressure from the board, they were refiled by another office. At that point, I realized that going to trial to restore my license would be futile. The trials are before an administrative law judge who renders an opinion. It is up to the board to make the final decision, and I knew what that would have been.

Having no funds left after having spent almost $500,000 in legal fees, and with no other options available to me, I agreed to surrender my license with the proviso that the misdemeanor charges would be removed. The deputy attorney general agreed to this request. After I signed the papers, not only did the board not honor the agreement, they forced the district attorney's office to change the charges from a misdemeanor to a felony. The settlement judge stated that in 20 years of sitting on the bench, he had never seen the medical review board pursue any doctor as viciously as they did me. A recent criticism of the board has been their inaction in going after doctors who have been sanctioned by hospitals for incompetence. The *Los Angeles Times* has published multiple articles about doctors who are killing patients by overprescribing narcotic medications. Many of these doctors have had multiple complaints filed against them, and yet the board failed to act. An example is a doctor in Santa Barbara who, despite multiple complaints filed to the board, caused the death of 410 of his patients via drug overdoses before he was finally arrested in early 2014 by the DEA. Is it possible that the medical review board is spending more energy eliminating doctors who they feel are practicing alternative medicine than they are investigating doctors who are killing patients with drugs or in surgery? Maybe it is time for this board to redefine its understanding of the "standard of care."

At present, the standard of care in medicine is dictated by the practices of the lowest common denominator of health care practitioners. They feel comfortable practicing within the cocoon of safety provided by state medical boards. These are traditional doctors, brainwashed by drug companies, who feel secure in giving out medications that often create more problems than the illnesses they are treating. They are reluctant to try anything "out of the box"; as a result, in my view, there has been no significant improvement in our approach to how we treat patients in the last 60 years. Doctors, for the most part, feel comfortable treating the symptoms of disease and give little thought to its causation. I do not find fault with these doctors, because this is how they were trained. However, the bottom line is that I can think of only a few medical conditions that we have eliminated in the 40 years I have been in practice. As a result, doctors still approach illnesses by giving out Band-Aids for hypertension, diabetes, depression, asthma, obesity, fibromyalgia, anxiety, insomnia, etc. The pharmaceutical industry keeps developing new drugs, but these have not led to an improvement in health care. There is certainly a financial benefit for drug companies and also for physicians—just plugging in the latest drug lets them see more patients in less time. However, it is not good for the patients, who are still not well and now have more side effects; it is not good for state and federal government, who are wasting billions of dollars on expensive medications and on the 400,000 hospitalizations per year for drug-related reactions. Insurance companies also pay for this inadequate approach, but they simply pass on the cost to the consumer, leading, of course, to higher premiums.

It seems that the primary function of state medical boards, such as the one in California, is to prevent any progress in medicine that can be harmful to the business of medicine. I can think of nothing more destructive to medical progress than to put traditional doctors in the role of evaluating alternative ideas. Except in extremely rare instances, the only significant breakthroughs in the treatment of cancer have been via alternative medicine. Of course, these therapies are viciously assaulted by our friends at the FDA, along with the help of medical boards.

As Voltaire said many years ago: "It is dangerous to be right in matters on which the established authorities are wrong."

There are continuous advances in every field of medicine—should they be eliminated or impeded (like stem cell therapy) because they are new? The field of bio-identical hormone therapy is basically unexplored territory. Doctors do not learn about it during their traditional training. Therefore, the standard of care should not be utilized when assessing natural hormone therapy, because "prudent" doctors have no knowledge of it. As long as pharmaceutical companies determine the rules of medicine, and the FDA and medical boards enforce them, it is unlikely that medical doctors will be allowed to follow the spirit and letter of the Hippocratic Oath, which they all swear to at the time of graduation from medical school.

EXCERPTS FROM THE HIPPOCRATIC OATH

I swear to fulfill, to the best of my ability and judgment, this covenant:

I will respect the hard-won scientific gains of those physicians in whose steps I walk, and gladly share knowledge as is mine with those who are to follow.

I will apply, for the benefit of the sick, all measures that are required, avoiding those twin traps of overtreatment and therapeutic nihilism. [This phrase is widely believed to be a translation of the Latin primum non nocere, *"first do no harm," which in fact does not appear in the Hippocratic Oath.]*

I will prevent disease whenever I can, for prevention is preferable to cure.

If I do not violate this oath, may I enjoy life and art, respected while I live and remembered with affection thereafter. May I always act so as to preserve the finest traditions of my calling and may I long experience the joy of healing those who seek my help.

The business of medicine thrives on disease and illness, not on wellness. This, in essence, is why there is no preventive medicine in this country, and why attempts are made from time to time to eliminate natural supplements from the marketplace. I suspect that the only reason that they have not been eliminated is that the ultimate aim of the pharmaceutical industry is to take over the nutriceutical companies. If that happens, supplements may only be available by prescription.

My hope is that, in some small way, this book will help change how medicine is practiced. I believe that once people become aware that there is a healthier way to address their health problems, a revolutionary change in medicine will occur.

MEAL PLAN TO LOWER ADRENALINE

The key to lowering adrenaline is to eliminate the underlying reason why the body is overproducing it. Since the brain uses more sugar than any other tissue in the body and must have sufficient fuel at all times, whenever the level of glucose in the brain is too low, the body releases adrenaline to raise the sugar level. The primary approach to managing adrenaline is to follow a meal plan designed to feed the body, and especially the brain, a steady supply of the proper amount and the right type of sugar (that is, from low-glycemic carbohydrates), along with using a bio-identical progesterone cream.

Because everyone's metabolism is different, there is no such thing as a one-size-fits-all meal plan. Thus the following meal plan should be treated as a set of guidelines, to be adjusted to the metabolic needs of each person's body and brain.

Even though this meal plan specifically addresses excess adrenaline, anyone who wants to eat healthfully can benefit from it. The plan will lower any excess adrenaline that may be contributing to stress. And because the meal plan keeps insulin production low, anyone with a weight problem can follow these guidelines to lose weight healthfully.

The meal plan is based on two key principles: eating or drinking the right type of carbohydrates with each meal and paying attention to the timing of meals. Low-glycemic carbohydrates provide the ideal fuel for the brain. High-glycemic foods—mostly refined carbohydrates such as white flour, white sugar, and products made with them—are digested quickly, which puts a lot of sugar into the bloodstream at once. This triggers the insulin–low sugar–adrenaline cycle that keeps adrenaline levels high. Low-glycemic foods—mostly unrefined foods, the kinds our bodies were designed to consume—are digested slowly, providing a steady supply of the right kinds of sugar into the bloodstream and then to the brain.

The timing of eating is important, especially for the creative brain, which seems to require feeding every three hours—a guideline that can actually work well for anyone. Thus the meal plan encourages eating smaller, even half-sized, portions four or five times throughout the day.

The brain, especially the creative brain, is working even while we are sleeping. So a light snack of a low-glycemic carbohydrate—such as green vegetables or brown rice or some sweet potato—just before bedtime can keep the brain from running out of fuel during the night.

Eating correctly is the single most important factor in lowering adrenaline. Results are often seen in just 24 hours.

MEAL PLAN GUIDELINES

WATER

If there is a magic liquid for weight loss and improved health, it is pure, clean water and lots of it. Water is the most abundant and important nutrient in the body. About 65 percent of the body is composed of water. Water regulates body temperature, transports nutrients, and builds tissues. It is required for joint lubrication, digestion, circulation, respiration, absorption, and excretion.

Not only do you need plenty of water for optimal health, you need water if you want to lose fat. If you are on a diet and dehydrated, you will burn muscle before you burn fat. The body is not able to burn fat efficiently without enough water. Your level of thirst is not a good indicator of your level of hydration. By the time your body registers the sensation of thirst, you are already somewhat dehydrated. Therefore, you should continue to drink water throughout the day, even when you are not thirsty. The secret is to not let yourself get dehydrated in the first place. If in doubt, drink more, not less.

To determine how much water you need to drink, divide your body weight in half. That number is the minimum number of ounces of water you should drink daily.

SUGAR

Avoid processed sugar and anything with sugar in it.

DAIRY

Avoid milk, ice cream, and flavored or sweetened yogurt. Use almond, rice, or coconut milk instead.

GRAINS

Avoid foods made with refined grains (white flour) such as pasta, breads, pastries, and many cereals. Choose products made with whole grains, such as multigrain or sprouted breads (Ezekiel is a good brand), high fiber cereals, vegetable pasta, and flax and rice crackers.

ALCOHOL

If you are serious about your health and you want maximum benefits from this program, alcoholic beverages should be eliminated. Alcohol is a potent diuretic. It draws water out of the cells and increases the loss of water through the kidneys. This can cause dehydration and its associated negative effects. If you are wanting to lose weight, avoid alcohol. In the body, the alcohol converts into sugar, so the body will burn the alcohol for fuel instead of burning fat.

VEGETABLES

A diet centered on fresh, raw, organic green vegetables (combined with lean proteins) is one of the best foundations for wellness (and for those trying to lose weight, an excellent way to get lean as quickly as possible). Green vegetables are the perfect sugar source for the brain. They are an excellent source of fibrous carbohydrates, contain relatively few calories, and it is virtually impossible to overeat them. Eat as many vegetables as you can. All varieties are good.

FRUITS

Fruits are excellent to include in a healthy diet. They provide a type of sugar called fructose, which is not utilized by the brain. The focus should be on low-glycemic fruits in order to lessen insulin production. Choose among: cherries (a small amount), oranges (not the juice), all berries, apricots, grapefruit, kiwis, plums, peaches, pears, green apples, and green bananas.

FIBER

Healthy, fiber-rich foods lower cholesterol and blood pressure, stabilize blood sugar levels, absorb toxins and poisons, and scrub the intestines, giving intestinal flora a place to colonize. Healthy choices include raw vegetables, nuts and seeds, oatmeal (steel cut is best), ground flaxseeds, and chia seeds.

PROTEIN

Healthy sources of protein include: lean beef, poultry (skinless chicken, turkey breast), fish (including sardines), and seafood, as well as legumes (peas and beans) of all kinds. Raw nuts (especially almonds), seeds (flax, sesame, sunflower, pumpkin, chia), and sprouts (sunflower, broccoli, alfalfa) are all good sources of protein. You may also include eggs or egg whites, cottage cheese, and high-protein whole grains (quinoa, millet, amaranth). The blue-green algae "superfoods" (sea greens, spirulina, chlorella) supply protein, as does nutritional yeast.

A vegetarian or vegan can get plenty of amino acids from the proteins available in vegetables, nuts, legumes, and superfoods.

FATS

Fats from plant sources are essential for hormonal balance, proper brain function, and weight loss. Some of the healthiest fats come from olives, olive oil, coconuts, coconut oil, avocados, nuts, fish, and fish oil.

GOOD (LOW-GLYCEMIC) CARBOHYDRATES

Be sure to eat plenty of complex carbohydrates. They are filling and provide long-term energy. These include mixed salads, all low-carbohydrate vegetables (including a variety of greens), sprouts, brown rice, steel-cut oatmeal, plain yogurt, kefir, yams, and sweet potatoes.

GREEN SMOOTHIES

A green smoothie is a blended drink consisting primarily of leafy greens like kale, collard greens, chard, spinach, lettuce, and wild greens, combined with fresh or frozen fruits like pineapple, mango, apple, pear, peaches, berries, kiwis, and green bananas. Smoothies offer an easily digested source of all the nutrients from fruits and vegetables, including calcium, protein, vitamins, and minerals. Drink one green smoothie daily. Several recipes for green smoothies are provided toward the end of this meal plan.

Sample Menu

The following are suggested meals for breakfast, lunch, and dinner. Experiment and eat a good variety of foods to prevent boredom.

Drink a full glass of water with the juice of half a fresh lemon when you first wake up.

Breakfast

- Drink a full glass of water before meal
- Apply progesterone one to three minutes before eating
- Scrambled eggs with sautéed onions and zucchini on a bed of baby spinach and sliced cucumbers

  Drink a full glass of water between breakfast and a morning snack.

Morning Snack

- Drink a full glass of water before snack
- Half of a green smoothie

  Drink a full glass of water between morning snack and lunch.

Lunch

- Drink a full glass of water before meal
- Apply progesterone one to three minutes before eating
- Make a generous green salad with lots of chopped

vegetables, sprinkled with nuts, seeds, or sprouts, topped lightly with herb-infused olive oil and lemon dressing

- Tuna fish or chicken added to the salad (optional)
- Only eat half of the salad

Drink a full glass of water between lunch and afternoon snack.

Afternoon Snack
- Drink a full glass of water before snack
- Eat the other half of the salad

Dinner
- Drink a full glass of water with the juice of half a fresh lemon before meal
- Apply progesterone one to three minutes before eating
- Poached salmon
- Half a cup brown rice
- Steamed vegetables

Evening Snack
- If you need an evening snack, enjoy celery sticks with almond butter

Bedtime Snack
If you tend to wake up during the night, try applying progesterone cream and eating something right before you go to bed, such as leftover vegetables from dinner, oatmeal, a green smoothie, or brown rice. You may also try a small amount of Greek yogurt.

The following are other ideas for meals. Mix and match and get creative!

Breakfast Ideas

Eggs, scrambled with green vegetables

No-crust spinach quiche

Oatmeal with flax seeds, blueberries, or strawberries

Soup

Brown rice cereal with flax seeds, cinnamon, and
slivered almonds

Plain Greek yogurt with berries, sliced apples, and
cinnamon

Lunch Ideas

Salad

Soup

Green smoothie or a protein drink with fruit

Burger or sandwich wrapped in
lettuce leaves instead of bread

Cottage cheese with berries or vegetables

Avocado, tomato, sprouts, and sliced cheese

(One possibility is to eat only half your lunch at lunchtime,
and have the other half as your afternoon snack three
hours later.)

Dinner Ideas

Lean meat, fish, or poultry

Green vegetables

Brown rice, brown rice pasta, or sweet potato

Beans

Soup or stew

Chili with lean meat or turkey

Stir-fry

Green smoothie

Snack Ideas

Raw vegetables dipped in nut butter or hummus

Deviled or boiled eggs

Tuna, chicken, or shrimp salad

Cottage cheese

Nuts and seeds

Sliced apples with cinnamon

Raw food bar or low-carbohydrate bar

Bowl of mixed fruit

Making Green Smoothies

When making green smoothies, keep it simple: Use only low-glycemic vegetables and fruits, plus water, along with some protein powder. Keep the ingredient list short. Keep the ingredients tasty so you continue to enjoy the benefits. Use organic ingredients as often as possible.

Fruit can be fresh or frozen. Frozen berries make a slushier smoothie. If you do not have a high-powered blender, avoid using all frozen fruit, or let frozen fruit thaw before blending. Avoid adding watermelon and other melons to smoothies; they are best digested on their own.

Greens can be purchased in bulk or in bags. Good greens to use include: mixed baby greens, spinach, kale, and romaine lettuce.

Peel, slice, and freeze green bananas, which are low in sugar, to use in smoothies.

Adding a protein powder, preferably a vegetable protein powder, to all of the following recipes is recommended. The protein balances the carbohydrates from the vegetables and thereby helps to control insulin. My office makes available a vegetable protein powder called Creative Meal Support that was specially formulated to help control adrenaline. Adding three tablespoons of extra virgin coconut oil to your smoothie is recommended. The following recipes will get you started. As you become familiar with making smoothies, feel free to experiment.

How to Make a Basic Green Smoothie

1. Pour one cup (or more) of water into a powerful blender.

2. Add protein powder.

3. Add chopped greens until the blender is full, and pulverize.

4. Add more greens to the blended greens and pulverize again.

5. Add cut up fruits in the combinations you think you will enjoy (suggested fruits are: apple, green banana, mango, and pineapple with mango) and pulverize again.

6. Add one to three tablespoons of coconut oil and briefly pulverize again.

Voila! You now have a basic green smoothie.

A tablespoon of freshly ground flaxseeds (buy whole seeds and grind in coffee grinder as needed) or whole chia seeds can be added to this smoothie. Adding a ripe avocado gives it a creamy texture and flavor. For a colder, frothier smoothie, add ice and blend.

Hint: If you or your family members or children are trying a smoothie for the first time, use very little greens and lots of fruit to avoid a strong greens flavor.

Do not add starchy vegetables to green smoothies. Starchy

vegetables include: carrots, beets, broccoli stems, zucchini, cauliflower, cabbage, brussels sprouts, eggplant, pumpkin, squash, okra, peas, corn, and green beans. Starchy vegetables combine poorly with fruit and may produce gas. Always rotate the green leaves that you add to your smoothies. Almost all greens contain minute amounts of alkaloids. Small quantities of alkaloids cannot hurt you and actually strengthen the immune system. However, if you keep consuming kale, spinach, or any other single green for many weeks without rotation, eventually the same types of alkaloids can accumulate in your body and cause unwanted symptoms of poisoning.

Green Smoothie Recipes

Easy Green Smoothie
8–10 oz water
2 handfuls of greens of choice
½ cup fruit of choice (low-glycemic)
1 tbsp of chia seeds or fresh ground flaxseed
vegetable protein powder

Tastes-Like-a-V-8 Smoothie
2 cups water
5 kale leaves
½ avocado
2 roma tomatoes
3 garlic cloves
Juice of ½ lime
½ tsp sea salt

Tropical Delight Smoothie

11 ounces water
1–2 handfuls of greens
Fruit from one young coconut
½ green papaya
1 cup pineapple
3–4 slices green banana

Very Veggie Blend

4 tomatoes
6 stalks celery
2 cucumbers
1 zucchini
Handful of chopped cilantro
1 small slice of red pepper
8–10 ounces of water

Kid-Friendly, Not Too Green Smoothie

3–4 slices of green banana
2 large rainbow chard leaves
1 heaping cup frozen cherries
Enough water to blend

Blue Smoothie

2–3 slices of frozen green banana
2 cups blueberries
2 apples
1 stick celery
4 huge leaves of kale
3 cups of water (or more to assist in blending)

This meal plan is fairly simple to follow and certainly not revolutionary. The take-home message is the importance of eating or drinking the right type of carbohydrates with each meal and eating small, frequent meals through the day, including right before bedtime if nighttime adrenaline is a problem.

APPENDIX B | GLYCEMIC INDEX

WHAT IS THE GLYCEMIC INDEX (GI)?*

The Glycemic Index (GI) is one the best tools for fat loss. It measures how quickly foods break down into sugar in your bloodstream. High glycemic foods turn into blood sugar very quickly. Starchy foods like potatoes are a good example. Potatoes have such a high GI rating, it's almost the same as eating table sugar. The glycemic index of green vegetables is zero because they convert into sugar slowly and thus stimulate little insulin production. Meat and most nuts contain no carbohydrates and thus stimulate no insulin production, so they also rate zero on the glycemic index scale.

WHAT IS THE GLYCEMIC LOAD (GL)?

The GI tells you how fast foods spike your blood sugar. But the GI won't tell you how much carbohydrate per serving you're getting. That's where the Glycemic Load (GL) is a great help. It measures the amount of carbohydrate in each serving of food. Foods with a glycemic load under 10 are good choices—these foods should be your first choice for carbs. Foods that fall between 10 and 20 on the glycemic load scale have a moderate effect on your blood sugar. Foods with a glycemic load above 20 will cause blood sugar and insulin spikes. Try to eat those foods sparingly.

* The information and chart provided here are reproduced with the permission of Al Sears, M.D. Please refer to his website for other excellent natural health, wellness, and anti-aging related information: www.alsearsmd.com.

FOOD	GI	Serving Size (g)	GL
CANDY/SWEETS			
Honey	87	2 tbs	17.9
Jelly Beans	78	1 oz	22
Snickers Bar	68	60g (½ bar)	23
Table Sugar	68	2 tsp	7
Strawberry Jam	51	2 tbs	10.1
Peanut M&M's	33	30g (1 oz)	5.6
Dove Dark Chocolate Bar	23	37g (1 oz)	4.4
BAKED GOODS & CEREALS			
Corn Bread	110	60g (1 piece)	30.8
French Bread	95	64g (1 slice)	29.5
Corn Flakes	92	28g (1 cup)	21.1
Corn Chex	83	30g (1 cup)	20.8
Rice Krispies	82	33g (1¼ cup)	23
Corn Pops	80	31g (1 cup)	22.4
Donut (lrg. glazed)	76	75g (1 donut)	24.3
Waffle (homemade)	76	75g (1 waffle)	18.7
Grape-Nuts	75	58g (½ cup)	31.5
Bran Flakes	74	29g (¾cup)	13.3
Graham Cracker	74	14g (2 squares)	8.1
Cheerios	74	30g (1 cup)	13.3
Kaiser Roll	73	57g (1 roll)	21.2
Bagel	72	*89g (¼ in.)	33
Corn Tortilla	70	24g (1 tortilla)	7.7
Melba Toast	70	12g (4 rounds)	5.6
Wheat Bread	70	28g (1 slice)	7.7
White Bread	70	25g (1 slice)	8.4

FOOD	GI	Serving Size (g)	GL
Kellogg's Special K	69	31g (1 cup)	14.5
Taco Shell	68	13g (1 med)	4.8
Angel Food Cake	67	28g (1 slice)	10.7
Croissant, Butter	67	57g (1 med)	17.5
Muselix	66	55g (⅔ cup)	23.8
Oatmeal, Instant	65	234g (1 cup)	13.7
Rye Bread, 100% Whole	65	32g (1 slice)	8.5
Rye Krisp Crackers	65	25 (1 wafer)	11.1
Raisin Bran	61	61g (1 cup)	24.4
Bran Muffin	60	113g (1 med)	30
Blueberry Muffin	59	113g (1 med)	30
Oatmeal	58	117g (½ cup)	6.4
Whole Wheat Pita	57	64g (1 pita)	17
Oatmeal Cookie	55	18g (1 large)	6
Popcorn	55	8g (1 cup)	2.8
Pound Cake, Sara Lee	54	30g (1 piece)	8.1
Vanilla Cake and Vanilla Frosting	42	64g (1 slice)	16
Pumpernickel Bread	41	26g (1slice)	4.5
Chocolate Cake w/ Chocolate Frosting	38	64g (1 slice)	12.5
BEVERAGES			
Gatorade Powder	78	16g (¾ scoop)	11.7
Cranberry Juice Cocktail	68	253g (1 cup)	24.5
Cola, Carbonated	63	370g (12oz can)	25.2
Orange Juice	57	249g (1 cup)	14.25
Hot Chocolate Mix	51	28g (1 packet)	11.7
Grapefruit Juice, Sweetened	48	250g (1 cup)	13.4

FOOD	GI	Serving Size (g)	GL
Pineapple Juice	46	250g (1 cup)	14.7
Soy Milk	44	245g (1 cup)	4
Apple Juice	41	248g (1 cup)	11.9
Tomato Juice	38	243g (1 cup)	3.4
LEGUMES			
Baked Beans	48	253g (1 cup)	18.2
Pinto Beans	39	171g (1 cup)	11.7
Lima Beans	31	241g (1 cup)	7.4
Chickpeas, Boiled	31	240g (1 cup)	13.3
Lentils	29	198g (1 cup)	7
Kidney Beans	27	256g (1 cup)	7
Soy Beans	20	172g (1 cup)	1.4
Peanuts	13	146g (1 cup)	1.6
VEGETABLES			
Potato	104	213g (1 med)	36.4
Parsnip	97	78g (½ cup)	11.6
Carrot, Raw	92	15g (1 large)	1
Beets, Canned	64	246g (½ cup)	9.6
Corn, Yellow	55	166g (1 cup)	61.5
Sweet Potato	54	133g (1 cup)	12.4
Yam	51	136g (1 cup)	16.8
Peas, Frozen	48	72g (½ cup)	3.4
Tomato	38	123g (1 med)	1.5
Broccoli, Cooked	0	78g (½ cup)	0
Cabbage, Cooked	0	75g (½ cup)	0
Celery, Raw	0	62g (1 stalk)	0

FOOD	GI	Serving Size (g)	GL
Cauliflower	0	100g (1 cup)	0
Green Beans	0	135g (1 cup)	0
Mushrooms	0	70g (1 cup)	0
Spinach	0	30g (1 cup)	0
FRUIT			
Watermelon	72	152g (1 cup)	7.2
Pineapple, Raw	66	155g (1 cup)	11.9
Cantaloupe	65	177g (1 cup)	7.8
Apricot, Canned in Light Syrup	64	253g (1 cup)	24.3
Raisins	64	43g (small box)	20.5
Papaya	60	140g (1 cup)	6.6
Peaches, Canned, Heavy Syrup	58	262g (1 cup)	28.4
Kiwi, w/ Skin	58	76g (1 fruit)	5.2
Fruit Cocktail, Drained	55	214g (1 cup)	19.8
Peaches, Canned, Light Syrup	52	251g (1 cup)	17.7
Banana	51	118g (1 med)	12.2
Mango	51	165g (1 cup)	12.8
Orange	48	140g (1 fruit)	7.2
Pears, Canned in Pear Juice	44	248g (1 cup)	12.3
Grapes	43	92g (1 cup)	6.5
Strawberries	40	152g (1 cup)	3.6
Apples, w/ Skin	39	138g (1 med)	6.2
Pears	33	166g (1 med)	6.9
Apricot, Dried	32	130g (1 cup)	23
Prunes	29	132g (1 cup)	34.2

FOOD	GI	Serving Size (g)	GL
Peach	28	98g (1 med)	2.2
Grapefruit	25	123g (½ fruit)	2.8
Plum	24	66g (1 fruit)	1.7
Sweet Cherries, Raw	22	117g (1 cup)	3.7
NUTS			
Cashews	22	---	0
Almonds	0	---	0
Hazelnuts	0	---	0
Macademia	0	---	0
Pecans	0	---	0
Walnuts	0		0
DAIRY			
Ice Cream (Lower Fat)	47	76g (½ cup)	9.4
Pudding	44	100g (½ cup)	8.4
Milk, Whole	40	244g (1 cup)	4.4
Ice Cream	38	72g (½ cup)	6
Yogurt, Plain	36	245g (1 cup)	6.1
MEAT/PROTEIN			
Beef	0	---	0
Chicken	0	---	0
Eggs	0	---	0
Fish	0	---	0
Lamb	0	---	0
Pork	0	---	0
Veal	0	---	0

FOOD	GI	Serving Size (g)	0
Deer–Venison	0	---	0
Elk	0	---	0
Buffalo	0	---	0
Rabbit	0	---	0
Duck	0	---	0
Ostrich	0	---	0
Shellfish	0	---	0
Lobster	0	---	0
Turkey	0	---	0
Ham	0	---	0

Follow these tips for Fat-Busting Meals:

• Avoid grains, including corn.

• Avoid potatoes and other white foods, like white rice, sugar, and salt.

• Try making protein the focus of each meal. It kicks your metabolism into higher gear. All meats, fish, and poultry are the real "guilt-free" foods. The protein will help you handle insulin better, build muscle, and repair tissue— all essential for staying lean and preventing diabetes.

• Snack on nuts and seeds. They are a good source of protein and have omega-3s.

• Avoid processed foods, trans fats, caffeine, and high fructose corn syrup. All increase insulin resistance.

• Choose vegetables that are low glycemic.

• Choose fruits such as berries and fruits that you can eat with the skin on.

• Eat a high protein breakfast every morning. It will stabilize your blood sugar and get you off to a good start.

THE MIRACLE OF BIO-IDENTICAL HORMONES

Winner of four national book awards, *The Miracle of Bio-Identical Hormones* is designed to help patients understand the importance of and rationale for hormone balancing. It includes patients' own stories of how their lives were transformed by following this approach to wellness. *The Miracle* is a best-selling hormone book in Europe and Asia.

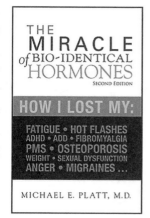

The Miracle of Bio-Identical Hormones by Michael E. Platt, M.D.
Clancy Lane Publishing, 2007.
219 pages. ISBN: 978-0977668328.

Available in Spanish:
El Milagro de las Hormonas Bio-Identicas,
Clancy Lane Publishing, 2007.

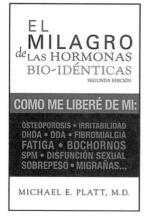

To order copies visit:
www.plattwellness.com
and click on the image of the book.

For wholesale orders of 10 or more ($12.50 each plus shipping), phone:
760-836-3232, or e-mail: questions@plattwellness.com.

Available in Germany as: *Die Hormon Revolution*

THE PLATT PROTOCOL FOR HORMONE BALANCING

Written for healthcare providers, *The Platt Protocol for Hormone Balancing* provides professionals with the information needed to incorporate the use of bio-identical hormones into their practice with confidence. It includes protocols for hormone usage to give to patients, as well as intake questionnaires. An entire chapter is dedicated to managing adrenaline.

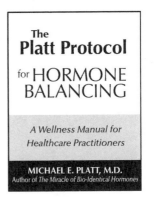

The Platt Protocol for Hormone Balancing
by Michael E. Platt, M.D.
Clancy Lane Publishing, 2012.
124 pages. ISBN: 978-0615649405.

To order copies visit:
www.plattwellness.com
and click on the image of the book.

INTRODUCING *Platt* PRO 5%

The strongest dose available without the need for a prescription!

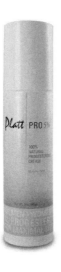

100% NATURAL PHARMACEUTICAL GRADE PROGESTERONE CREAM

Platt Pro 5% is a natural, bio-identical progesterone cream specially formulated by Dr. Platt to provide maximal effectiveness. The large, 3–ounce pump container provides 50 mg of progesterone per pump. This is the initial dose that Dr. Platt recommends.

Platt Pro 5% is available at a wholesale price for practitioners interested in providing their clients or patients with the benefits of progesterone.

A brochure provided with each order explains the benefits of progesterone as well as the most effective way to use it.

BALANCING • FOR MEN+WOMEN OF ALL AGES
BIO-IDENTICAL PROGESTERONE CREAM
FORMULATED FOR MAXIMAL EFFECTIVENESS

Order online at: plattwellness.com, or call: 760.836.3232

**For further information about
Dr. Platt and his work:**

website: www.plattwellness.com

e-mail: questions@plattwellness.com

phone: 760-836-3232